THE YOGA CURE:

30-Day Guide to Relief from Stress, Pain, and Fatigue

Discover the Power of Yoga to Heal Your Body and Recharge Your Life

Diana Shaw

To my family, whose unwavering support and love have been my foundation,

To my friends, who have inspired and encouraged me every step of the way,

And to all the dreamers and doers, who strive for success and never give up,

This book is dedicated to you.

May it be a guide and a source of inspiration on your journey to achieving your dreams.

With heartfelt gratitude.

ABSTRACT

The Yoga Cure: 30-Day Guide to Relief from Stress, Pain, and Fatigue is a comprehensive, accessible guide to using yoga as a tool for physical and mental well-being. This book offers a structured 30-day program designed to relieve stress, alleviate chronic pain, and combat fatigue through the transformative power of yoga. Each week focuses on different aspects of healing, starting with foundational practices that build body awareness and mindfulness, followed by techniques to release tension, manage pain in specific areas, and restore energy. The book combines gentle yoga poses, restorative breathwork, and mental techniques that promote relaxation, balance, and vitality. With a focus on individualized practices and ongoing self-care, *The Yoga Cure* empowers readers to personalize their yoga journey, offering tools to integrate these healing practices into their daily lives. The book is an ideal resource for anyone seeking a holistic approach to managing stress, pain, and fatigue, providing practical tools to create lasting health and well-being.

TABLE OF CONTENT

Introduction

Overview of Yoga as a Healing Modality

Yoga is an ancient practice that has been passed down for thousands of years, originating in India as a way to cultivate physical, mental, and spiritual well-being. Derived from the Sanskrit word yuj, which means "to yoke" or "to unite," yoga is a method of uniting the body, mind, and spirit to create a sense of inner harmony. Historically, yoga was practiced as a path to self-realization, a way to understand one's connection to the universe and transcend suffering. Over time, the practice evolved, and different schools of yoga emerged, each with unique philosophies, techniques, and focuses, such as Hatha, Ashtanga, and Kundalini.

In the modern world, yoga has become a powerful therapeutic tool for healing and wellness. While yoga is commonly associated with physical postures (asana), it is a multi-faceted practice that includes breathwork (pranayama), meditation (dhyana), and ethical principles (yamas and niyamas). Together, these elements foster a balanced, holistic approach to health. Today, yoga is recognized not only as an effective physical workout but as a healing modality that addresses the complex relationship between the mind and body.

The benefits of yoga are well-documented and far-reaching, addressing three critical aspects of human health: the mind, body, and spirit. For the mind, yoga cultivates mental clarity, reduces stress, and fosters mindfulness. For the body, yoga builds strength, flexibility, and endurance, and supports joint health and overall circulation. For the spirit, yoga helps practitioners connect with their inner selves, fostering a sense of peace, gratitude, and purpose.

How Stress, Pain, and Fatigue Affect Our Lives

Chronic stress, physical pain, and fatigue are widespread issues in today's fast-paced world, affecting millions of people's quality of life. Each of these issues can have severe impacts on both mental and physical health, and they often interconnect, creating a cycle of discomfort and exhaustion that can be challenging to break.

Chronic Stress: Stress is a natural response to challenges or perceived threats, but when it becomes chronic, it can lead to a range of health issues. Chronic stress increases cortisol levels, which can disrupt sleep, impair immune function, and increase the risk of heart disease. It also causes muscle tension, poor digestion, and heightened sensitivity to pain. Emotionally, prolonged stress can lead to anxiety, depression, and burnout, affecting personal relationships and overall well-being. In response to chronic stress, the body remains in a constant state of alert, which, over time, drains energy and disrupts normal physiological functioning.

Physical Pain: Pain, especially chronic pain, often results from injury, inflammation, poor posture, or prolonged tension in muscles and joints. Pain affects physical abilities and can interfere with daily activities, limiting mobility and causing frustration and emotional distress. Pain can also be exacerbated by stress, creating a feedback loop where pain intensifies stress, which in turn increases the perception of pain. This cycle affects emotional well-being, leading to feelings of helplessness, depression, and even isolation.

Fatigue: Fatigue, whether physical or mental, is an overwhelming feeling of exhaustion and lack of energy. Chronic fatigue can stem from various sources, including sleep disorders, poor diet, stress, and a lack of physical activity. Fatigue affects focus, mood, and productivity, and it can impair the body's ability to heal and regulate itself. The exhaustion of chronic fatigue often makes it challenging to engage in physical activities, which in turn leads to muscle weakness, poor circulation, and a reduced sense of vitality.

By understanding the intricate ways that stress, pain, and fatigue affect our lives, it becomes clear why a holistic practice like yoga can be so effective in addressing these interconnected issues. Yoga provides tools for releasing tension, improving physical strength and flexibility, and nurturing a calmer state of mind, which can gradually break the cycle of stress, pain, and fatigue.

The Science Behind Yoga's Healing Power

The healing power of yoga lies in its ability to activate the body's natural processes of relaxation, regeneration, and resilience. Scientific studies have shown that yoga influences the nervous system, the immune system, and mental health in profound ways.

Nervous System: Yoga has a significant impact on the autonomic nervous system, which controls the body's involuntary responses. Through controlled breathing, movement, and meditation, yoga stimulates the parasympathetic nervous system (often referred to as the "rest and digest" system). This activation reduces the "fight or flight" response driven by the sympathetic nervous system, lowering heart rate, blood pressure, and stress hormone levels. Regular yoga practice can help recalibrate the body's response to stress, making it easier to manage tension and anxiety in daily life. This calming effect on the nervous system also improves sleep quality, boosts energy levels, and promotes emotional resilience.

Immune System: Chronic stress weakens the immune system, leaving the body vulnerable to illness and inflammation. Yoga's stress-reducing effects enhance immune function, lowering inflammation markers and improving the body's ability to defend itself against infection. Specific yoga poses and breathing techniques increase circulation, promote lymphatic drainage, and aid in detoxification, which helps the body fight off pathogens more effectively.

Mental Health: Yoga's emphasis on mindfulness and breathing helps to calm the mind, improve focus, and promote emotional regulation. Yoga has been shown to reduce symptoms of anxiety, depression, and PTSD by increasing the release of "feel-good" neurotransmitters, such as serotonin and dopamine. Meditation practices in yoga encourage a deeper understanding of thought patterns, making it easier to let go of negative mental habits and cultivate a sense of inner peace. Practitioners often experience improved self-esteem, a positive outlook on life, and an increased ability to cope with stressors.

Yoga's impact on the nervous system, immune system, and mental health has led to its recognition as an effective complementary therapy for managing stress, pain, and fatigue, providing benefits that extend beyond physical fitness.

How to Use This Book

This book is structured as a 30-day program designed to progressively guide you through a journey of relief and revitalization. Each week is dedicated to a specific focus area to help you build strength, flexibility, and mindfulness.

- **Week 1: Building Awareness and Foundations** focuses on cultivating a connection with your body and breath, introducing foundational poses and breathwork techniques to support relaxation.
- **Week 2: Releasing Stress and Tension** includes restorative poses and mindful breathing to release mental and physical stress, helping you identify and relieve areas of chronic tension.
- **Week 3: Managing Pain with Targeted Yoga Practices** guides you through poses and sequences specifically designed for pain relief, addressing common areas of discomfort such as the back, neck, shoulders, and hips.
- **Week 4: Boosting Energy and Combating Fatigue** introduces energizing routines and mindfulness techniques that recharge your body and spirit, giving you tools to maintain vitality and avoid burnout.

Each chapter contains step-by-step instructions for poses and sequences, tips for proper alignment, and modifications to suit all levels. Alongside physical practice, you will find breathwork exercises and mindfulness prompts to deepen your experience and foster a sense of calm and clarity. Journaling exercises are provided to help you reflect on your journey, track your progress, and recognize the changes you feel.

As you follow this 30-day guide, remember that yoga is a personal journey, and each individual's path may look different. Approach the practice with curiosity and patience, allowing yourself the time to connect with your body, observe your mind, and embrace the restorative benefits yoga has to offer. Whether you're new to yoga or looking to deepen an existing practice, this program provides a structured, supportive path to help you relieve stress, manage pain, and rejuvenate your energy, one day at a time.

Week 1: Building Awareness and Foundations

Goal

In the first week, the focus is on building awareness, laying down the physical and mental foundations for a successful yoga practice. This week introduces you to foundational poses, simple breathing techniques, and mindful practices that will help you connect with your body and breath. These essential elements establish the core skills you'll need as you progress through the program, creating a foundation for healing and relaxation.

Chapter 1: The Mind-Body Connection

Explanation of the Mind-Body Relationship and Its Role in Healing

The mind and body are interconnected in complex ways, each influencing the health and functioning of the other. This relationship is the foundation of holistic healing practices, including yoga, which recognizes that physical and mental states are not separate but rather deeply intertwined. When we experience mental stress, for example, our bodies often respond with muscle tension, digestive issues, and elevated heart rates. Conversely, physical discomfort or chronic pain can heighten anxiety, depression, and frustration.

Yoga operates on the principle that healing occurs most effectively when both mind and body are in harmony. By tuning into the body and becoming aware of our physical sensations, we can better understand our emotional states. The practice of yoga encourages this awareness, helping practitioners recognize and release physical tension, become mindful of thoughts and emotions, and, ultimately, foster a sense of peace and balance.

Through consistent practice, yoga cultivates mindfulness—the ability to observe one's thoughts and sensations without judgment. This awareness allows us to break habitual cycles of stress and negative thinking, fostering resilience and emotional balance. The mind-body connection promoted in yoga is a powerful tool for healing because it enables us to understand our bodies' signals, giving us insight into the needs of both our physical and mental selves. When we honor these signals, we empower ourselves to move toward better health and well-being.

The Importance of Breathing, Body Awareness, and Alignment

Breathing (Pranayama)

Breath, or prana, is the life force that sustains our body and mind. In yoga, breathing exercises, known as pranayama, are used to regulate energy, calm the mind, and prepare the body for physical movement. Pranayama helps us connect to the present moment, as each breath becomes an anchor that quiets the mind and draws our focus inward. Breathing with awareness also activates the parasympathetic nervous system, promoting a state of relaxation, slowing the heart rate, and lowering blood pressure.

In yoga, breath serves several roles:

- **Focus and Grounding**: Slow, controlled breathing quiets the mind, bringing a sense of calm and grounding.
- **Release of Tension**: Exhaling allows for the conscious release of tension from the body, both physically and mentally.
- **Energy Management**: Breathing exercises can energize the body, preparing it for physical movement, or calm the body in preparation for rest and relaxation.

Body Awareness

Body awareness, often referred to as proprioception, is our ability to sense the position and movement of our bodies. Practicing yoga enhances body awareness by helping us notice how our muscles, joints, and breath feel in each posture. This awareness not only helps us execute poses more safely and effectively but also increases our connection to our physical self.

As we become more attuned to our body's signals, we learn to detect areas of tightness, misalignment, or fatigue, which can offer valuable insights into our mental and emotional state. For example, tension in the shoulders and neck might indicate unresolved stress, while discomfort in the hips could signify stored emotional strain. Body awareness fosters self-compassion, allowing us to listen to our body's needs, respect its limits, and find joy in its capabilities.

Alignment

Alignment refers to the proper positioning of the body in each yoga posture. Practicing alignment helps prevent injury, promotes balance, and allows the body's energy to flow freely. Each yoga pose has an optimal alignment to ensure that muscles, joints, and bones work together harmoniously. Proper alignment is essential for gaining the full benefit of each pose, as it creates stability, promotes even stretching, and minimizes strain on vulnerable areas.

In the context of the mind-body connection, alignment is not just physical; it is a practice of mindfulness and awareness. As you align your body, you bring focus to each movement, each muscle, and each breath. This focused attention creates a meditative state, calming the mind and building a strong connection between mind and body.

Introduction to Pranayama (Breathing Exercises) for Relaxation and Energy

Breathing exercises, or pranayama, are a central component of yoga, offering a direct way to influence the mind-body connection. By controlling the breath, we can calm the nervous system, reduce stress, and bring renewed energy into the body.

Here are three introductory pranayama techniques that are especially effective for relaxation and energy management:

1. **Diaphragmatic Breathing (Deep Belly Breathing)**

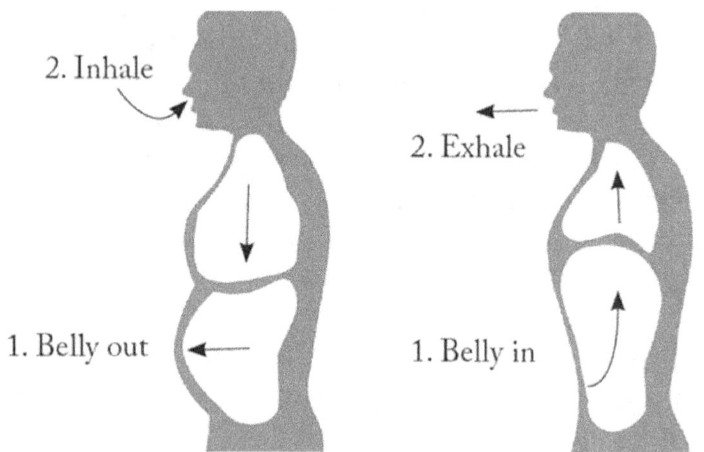

- o **Purpose**: To promote relaxation, reduce stress, and enhance body awareness.
- o **Practice**: Place one hand on your chest and the other on your abdomen. Inhale deeply through your nose, allowing your belly to expand as you fill your lungs with air.

Exhale slowly, feeling your belly fall. Focus on making your inhales and exhales long and smooth.

- o **Benefits**: Activates the diaphragm, increases oxygen intake, and calms the nervous system, encouraging a state of relaxation.

2. **Ujjayi Breath (Ocean Breath)**

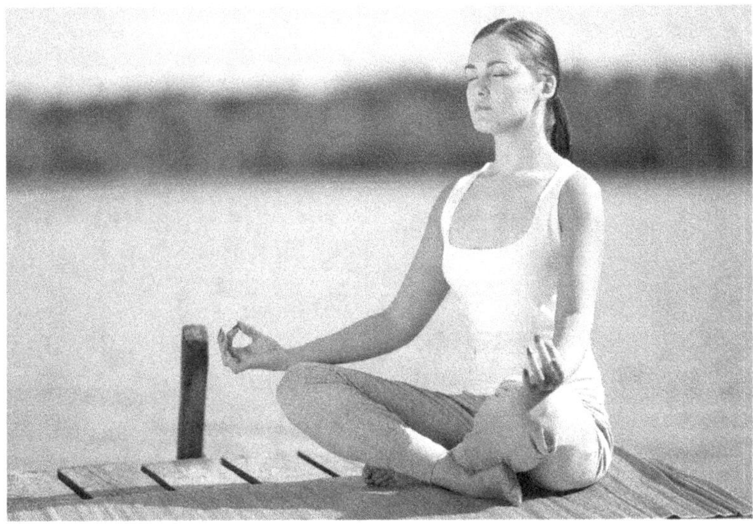

- o **Purpose**: To create a sense of calm and focus, ideal for use during physical practice.
- o **Practice**: With your mouth closed, inhale deeply through your nose, constricting the back of your throat slightly to create a soft "ocean wave" sound. Exhale through the nose, maintaining the constriction to create a steady rhythm.

- **Benefits**: Balances energy, calms the mind, and promotes a meditative focus during movement, making it easier to connect breath and body.

3. **4-7-8 Breath**

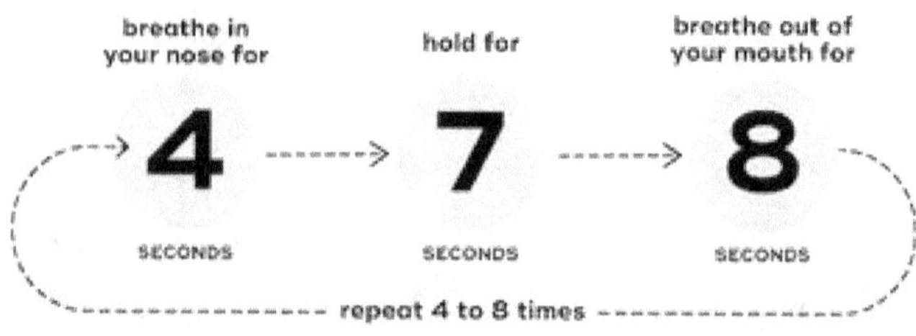

- **Purpose**: To quickly calm the mind and body, especially helpful for relieving anxiety.
- **Practice**: Inhale through the nose for a count of 4, hold the breath for a count of 7, and then exhale slowly through the mouth for a count of 8. Repeat this cycle several times, maintaining a relaxed posture.
- **Benefits**: Slows the heart rate, reduces tension, and promotes relaxation by activating the body's relaxation response.

In practicing pranayama, remember that breath is not only a physiological process but also a powerful tool for self-awareness and transformation. Each breath is an opportunity to cultivate mindfulness, bringing you closer to the state of peace and balance that lies at the heart of the mind-body connection. As you move through each yoga pose, let your breath be your guide, helping you stay present, release tension, and connect more deeply with your body.

Reflection Exercise:

- At the end of this week, take time to journal about your experience with the mind-body connection. What sensations did you notice in your body? How did focused breathing affect your state of mind? Write down any shifts in your awareness or feelings of calm.

This chapter lays the groundwork for a mindful yoga practice that will be built upon in the coming weeks. By learning to connect with your body, align your movements, and breathe with intention, you are establishing the essential tools for healing, growth, and transformation.

Chapter 2: Foundational Poses for Stability and Strength

Overview

In this chapter, you'll be introduced to foundational yoga poses that will form the building blocks of your practice. These poses—Mountain, Child's Pose, Cat-Cow, and Downward-Facing Dog—are simple yet powerful, emphasizing alignment, balance, and flexibility. Practicing these postures regularly can help you build stability and strength, which are essential for safe movement and proper form. You'll also learn modifications to suit all levels, as well as gentle routines you can incorporate into your mornings and evenings to support a consistent, balanced practice.

Foundational Poses

1. Mountain Pose (Tadasana)

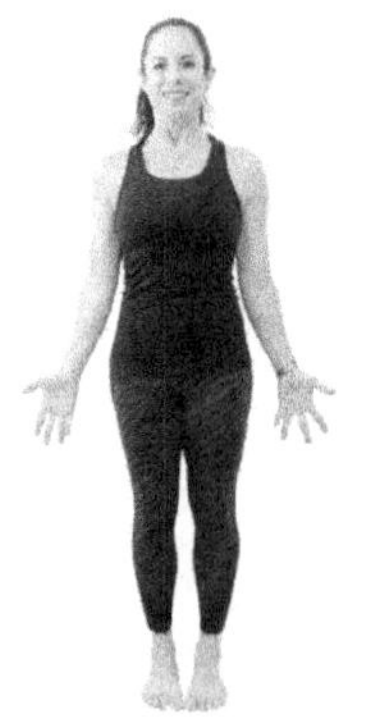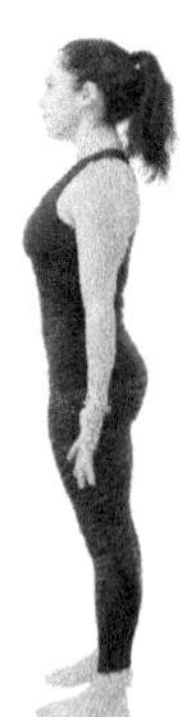

- **Purpose**: To develop balance, improve posture, and promote body awareness.
- **How to Practice**:
  - Stand with your feet hip-width apart, pressing evenly into the ground with all parts of your feet.
  - Lift your toes briefly to engage the arches of your feet, then relax them back onto the mat.
  - Lengthen through your spine, roll your shoulders back, and allow your arms to rest at your sides with palms facing forward.
  - Engage your core slightly, tucking your pelvis to avoid arching in the lower back.
  - Breathe deeply, feeling the connection of your feet to the earth and the extension through the crown of your head.
- **Alignment Tips**: Keep weight distributed evenly, avoid locking the knees, and maintain a neutral pelvis.
- **Modification**: Stand with feet slightly apart if you need more stability. If balance is challenging, practice with your back against a wall for support.

2. Child's Pose (Balasana)

- **Purpose**: To gently stretch the hips, thighs, and lower back while promoting relaxation and grounding.
- **How to Practice**:

- o Start on your knees, bringing your big toes together and knees apart.
  - o Sit back on your heels and fold forward, extending your arms in front of you or resting them alongside your body.
  - o Let your forehead rest on the mat, taking slow, deep breaths.
  - o Soften into the posture with each exhale, allowing tension to release from the shoulders and lower back.
- **Alignment Tips**: Keep your hips as close to your heels as comfortable and allow your spine to lengthen.
- **Modification**: Place a cushion or blanket between your hips and heels if you feel discomfort. You can also rest your head on a block or stack your fists to support your neck.

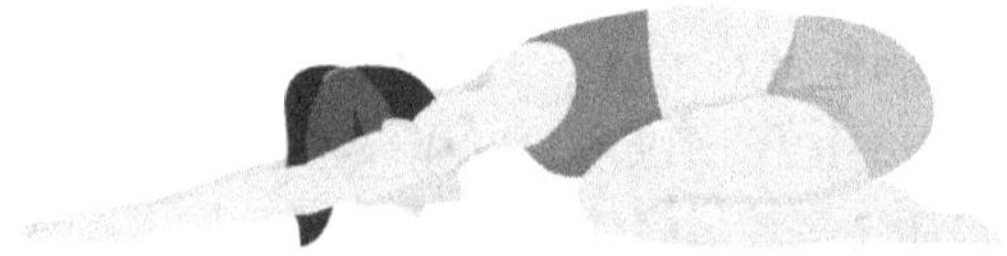

3. Cat-Cow Pose (Marjaryasana-Bitilasana)

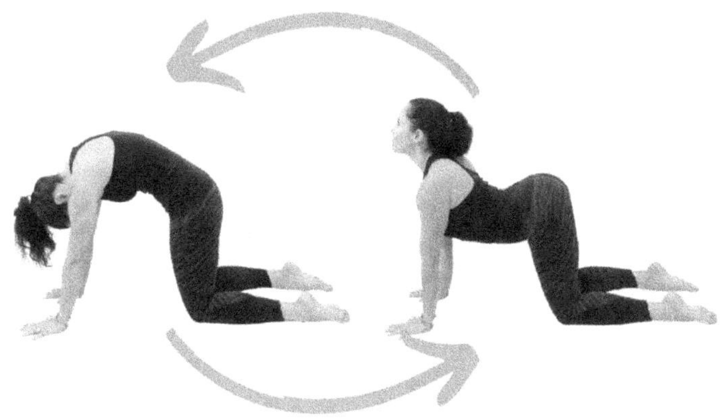

- **Purpose**: To warm up the spine, release tension, and improve flexibility in the back and neck.
- **How to Practice**:
    - Begin on all fours, with your wrists aligned under your shoulders and knees under your hips.
    - Inhale as you arch your spine, lifting your tailbone and head (Cow Pose).
    - Exhale as you round your spine, drawing your navel in and tucking your chin toward your chest (Cat Pose).
    - Continue moving slowly with your breath, flowing between the two poses.

- **Alignment Tips**: Keep movements smooth and intentional, focusing on coordinating breath with movement.
- **Modification**: If you experience wrist discomfort, place a folded blanket under your hands or come down onto your forearms.

4. Downward-Facing Dog (Adho Mukha Svanasana)

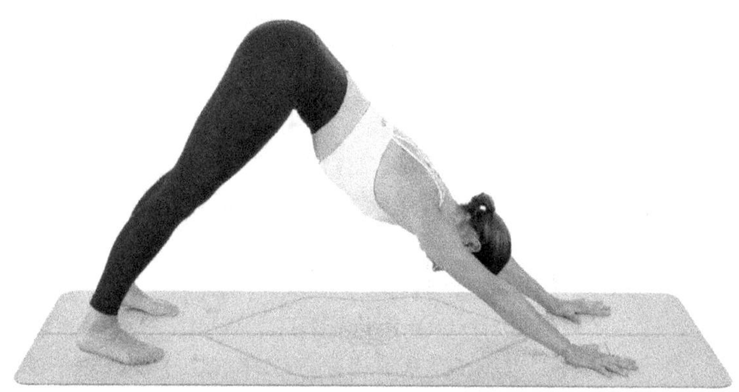

- **Purpose**: To build strength in the arms, shoulders, and legs while providing a gentle stretch to the hamstrings, calves, and back.
- **How to Practice**:
  - Begin on all fours. Tuck your toes, lift your hips, and straighten your legs, forming an inverted V shape.
  - Press firmly into your hands, especially through the index finger

and thumb, to avoid strain on the wrists.
  - o Lengthen your spine and allow your heels to move toward the mat, bending your knees slightly if needed.
  - o Keep your neck relaxed and gaze slightly forward or down, with ears aligned between your arms.
- **Alignment Tips**: Focus on lengthening the spine rather than forcing the heels to the floor. Keep your shoulders broad and avoid locking the elbows.
- **Modification**: Bend your knees to make the pose more accessible if you have tight hamstrings or lower back discomfort. You can also use a wall for support, pressing your hands against the wall while keeping a neutral spine.

Emphasis on Proper Alignment and Modifications for All Levels

Alignment is essential for avoiding injury and maximizing the benefits of each pose. Practicing with proper alignment ensures that your muscles and joints work together in a balanced way, reducing unnecessary strain. As you work through these foundational poses, pay close attention to your form, and adjust as needed based on your body's needs.

Key Alignment Tips:

- **Maintain a Neutral Spine**: Avoid excessive rounding or arching, and engage your core to support your back.
- **Distribute Weight Evenly**: In standing poses like Mountain, keep weight balanced across all four corners of the feet. In poses like Downward-Facing Dog, distribute weight evenly between hands and feet.
- **Modify as Needed**: Use props like blocks, blankets, and straps to make poses more accessible. Modifications are a valuable tool for creating a sustainable practice that works with your body.

Examples of Modifications:

- Use a folded blanket under the knees in Child's Pose to ease pressure.
- Bend your knees in Downward-Facing Dog to avoid straining the lower back or hamstrings.
- Practice against a wall for balance assistance in Mountain Pose or Downward-Facing Dog.

Gentle Routines for Morning and Evening

Incorporating yoga into your morning and evening routines can set a positive tone for the day and help you wind down at night. Here are short sequences you can practice to ground and refresh yourself.

Morning Routine (10-15 minutes)

- **Mountain Pose (Tadasana)**: Begin standing, grounding yourself and connecting with your breath.
- **Cat-Cow Flow (Marjaryasana-Bitilasana)**: Warm up your spine, moving mindfully with your breath.
- **Downward-Facing Dog (Adho Mukha Svanasana)**: Transition into Downward Dog, taking a few breaths here to stretch and energize the body.
- **Child's Pose (Balasana)**: End with Child's Pose, focusing on setting a calm, positive intention for the day.

Benefits: This routine gently awakens the body, stretches muscles, and boosts circulation, preparing you for the day ahead.

Evening Routine (10-15 minutes)

- **Child's Pose (Balasana)**: Start in Child's Pose, breathing deeply and letting go of the day's tension.
- **Cat-Cow Flow (Marjaryasana-Bitilasana)**: Loosen the spine and relieve any tightness accumulated from sitting or daily activities.
- **Downward-Facing Dog (Adho Mukha Svanasana)**: Transition into Downward

Dog, staying here for a few breaths to release the back and hamstrings.

- **Seated Forward Fold (Paschimottanasana)**: From a seated position, gently fold forward over your legs to stretch the back and legs, promoting relaxation.
- **Savasana (Corpse Pose)**: Lie flat on your back, arms at your sides, and allow yourself to fully relax, focusing on slow, steady breathing.

Benefits: This evening sequence calms the mind, releases muscle tension, and prepares the body for restful sleep.

- **Reflection**: At the end of this week, journal about your experience with the foundational poses. Did you notice any changes in your strength, stability, or flexibility? How did focusing on alignment and using modifications affect your practice?

By focusing on these foundational poses, you are creating a solid base for a safe and effective yoga practice. As you deepen your awareness of alignment, balance, and modifications, you'll feel more confident and prepared to move forward in your yoga journey.

Chapter 3: Establishing a Daily Routine

Overview

One of the most rewarding aspects of yoga is its adaptability; it can be practiced almost anywhere and can fit into even the busiest schedules. In this chapter, you'll learn how to incorporate yoga into your daily life, creating a routine that feels manageable and sustainable. We'll cover strategies for finding time in your day, tips for setting up a dedicated yoga space, and the benefits of journaling to track your progress and observe any changes in your energy levels, mood, and overall well-being.

How to Incorporate Daily Practice into a Busy Life

A daily yoga practice doesn't have to be lengthy to be effective. Consistency is more valuable than duration—10 to 20 minutes a day can provide significant benefits if practiced regularly. Here are some strategies to make yoga a seamless part of your day, even if you have a busy schedule.

1. Choose a Time That Works for You

- Morning and evening are often the best times to practice, but the ideal time is whenever you can commit to consistently. Consider your natural energy levels: some

people enjoy the calm of morning yoga, while others prefer a relaxing session before bed.
- Set an intention to show up, even for just a few minutes. It's better to practice a short routine daily than a longer routine sporadically.

2. Start Small and Build Gradually

- Begin with 5-10 minutes a day, which is easier to commit to and helps build a habit. Once you're comfortable with this, you can gradually extend the duration.
- If you're short on time, focus on a few poses that bring the most benefits for your body and mind, such as Downward-Facing Dog to stretch and energize, or Child's Pose for relaxation.

3. Incorporate Mindful Movement During the Day

- Yoga doesn't have to be limited to a mat; you can incorporate mindful movement and breathing into daily activities. Take a few deep breaths while waiting in line, stretch gently at your desk, or do a few simple poses during a break.
- Practicing mindfulness throughout your day supports your yoga routine by reinforcing the mind-body connection and stress relief.

4. Use a Reminder System

- Set reminders on your phone or calendar for your practice time. You could also associate your practice with an existing habit, like brushing your teeth, to make it easier to remember.
- Consider using a yoga app or a tracker to log your practice, which can help reinforce your routine.

5. Be Flexible and Patient

- Your routine doesn't have to be perfect. Life can be unpredictable, and it's okay if some days are busier than others. A flexible attitude toward your practice will help you maintain a sense of progress without unnecessary pressure.
- Practice self-compassion. Yoga is a journey, not a destination, and it's normal for your practice to change with your schedule and energy levels.

Tips for Setting Up a Yoga Space at Home

Creating a dedicated space for your yoga practice can make it easier to establish a routine and enhance the quality of your sessions. Here are some tips for designing a calm, inviting yoga space at home, even if you're working with limited space.

1. Find a Quiet, Distraction-Free Area

- Look for a spot in your home that's free from distractions, ideally where you won't be interrupted. Even a small area in your bedroom or living room can work as long as it allows you to stretch comfortably.
- If you share your home with others, let them know about your practice time so they can respect your need for quiet during those moments.

2. Create a Calming Atmosphere

- Use soft lighting, and consider adding candles, incense, or essential oils to create a calming environment. Scents like lavender, chamomile, or eucalyptus can enhance relaxation.
- If you're able, incorporate elements from nature, such as a plant, small stones, or a water fountain, to connect with the grounding qualities of nature.

3. Add Comfortable, Supportive Props

- A good-quality yoga mat is a foundational piece of equipment that can make a big difference in your practice. Choose one with enough cushioning to protect your joints.
- Consider adding props like a bolster, blocks, or a strap to support you in poses and help with modifications. Blankets and

cushions can also be helpful for comfort and relaxation.

4. Personalize Your Space

- Personal touches can make your yoga space more inviting. Place items that inspire you—whether it's a favorite book, photo, or motivational quote—near your space as reminders of your intention and commitment to wellness.
- You can also keep a journal and pen nearby, which can make it easier to record reflections after practice.

5. Make It Multi-Purpose If Needed

- If you don't have a dedicated space, store your yoga mat and props in an accessible place and roll them out when it's time to practice. Keeping your space tidy after each session makes it easy to return to practice the next day.
- Consider using a corner of your living room, a hallway, or even a quiet outdoor spot if the weather permits.

Creating a Journal to Track Feelings, Energy Levels, and Changes

Journaling is a powerful tool that can enhance your yoga practice by helping you observe patterns, progress, and insights gained through regular practice. In addition to tracking physical progress, a journal can help you become more mindful of shifts in your mental and emotional well-being.

1. Reflect on Physical Sensations and Energy Levels

- After each practice, take a few minutes to write down how your body feels. Note any areas of tightness, relief, or strength, as well as any shifts in flexibility.
- Track your energy levels before and after practice, noticing any changes. Are you feeling more refreshed or relaxed? This can help you understand which practices benefit you most.

2. Observe Emotional and Mental Shifts

- Yoga is as much a mental practice as a physical one, and your journal can help you observe emotional changes that occur over time. For example, you may notice feelings of calm, gratitude, or reduced stress after practicing.
- Note any mental clarity, focus, or sense of peace that emerges during or after yoga. These reflections can deepen your understanding of how yoga supports your emotional health.

3. Track Your Progress and Challenges

- Use your journal to celebrate small victories, like improving your flexibility or finding ease in a particular pose. Acknowledging these achievements reinforces positive change and motivates you to continue.
- If you encounter challenges or poses that feel difficult, write them down without judgment. Over time, you may notice these areas evolve as you build strength and flexibility.

4. Set Intentions and Goals

- Each week or month, set a new intention or goal for your practice, such as focusing on mindfulness, developing strength, or simply practicing consistently. Writing down your intentions reinforces your commitment and helps you stay focused.
- Review these intentions regularly, adjusting them as needed. Intentions can help keep your practice aligned with your personal goals and values.

5. Monthly Reflections

- At the end of each month, review your entries to see how your practice has impacted your physical, mental, and emotional well-being. This reflection helps you understand your journey more deeply and encourages gratitude for the progress you've made.

- Reflect on any changes in your stress, pain, or fatigue levels and how yoga has supported you in managing these areas. Noticing these shifts will reinforce the positive role yoga plays in your life.

Reflection: As you wrap up this chapter, take time to set up your journal, choose your practice space, and decide on a time that feels right for your daily practice. Track your experiences over the coming days, noting any shifts in your mindset, body, or energy levels.

By establishing a dedicated space, setting realistic intentions, and journaling your journey, you'll be well-equipped to maintain a fulfilling yoga practice that fits your life. This daily commitment becomes an investment in your well-being, helping you foster a stable, nurturing relationship with yoga that supports your healing and growth.

Week 2: Releasing Stress and Tension

Goal: Focus on relieving mental and physical stress, with restorative poses and breathwork.

Chapter 4: Understanding Stress and Its Impact on the Body

Overview

Stress affects the body and mind in complex ways, often showing up physically long before we realize its presence emotionally or mentally. In this chapter, we'll explore how stress manifests in the body, including symptoms like muscle tension, headaches, and digestive issues. You'll also learn practical tools to identify and address the sources of stress in your daily life, empowering you to manage stress more effectively and improve your overall well-being.

How Stress Manifests Physically

When we experience stress, our bodies respond with a series of physiological changes known as the "fight-or-flight" response. This response is beneficial in short bursts, helping us stay alert and responsive. However, chronic stress keeps our bodies in this heightened state, which can lead to lasting physical symptoms and health challenges.

1. Muscle Tension and Pain

- **How It Manifests**: Stress often causes the muscles, especially those in the neck, shoulders, and back, to tense up. This tension can lead to stiffness, soreness, and even chronic pain.
- **Long-Term Effects**: Persistent muscle tension can contribute to more severe issues, such as tension headaches, migraines, and even posture-related pain over time.
- **Yoga's Role**: Gentle stretching, breathwork, and restorative poses help release muscle tension, reduce pain, and promote relaxation in these commonly affected areas.

2. Headaches and Migraines

- **How It Manifests**: Stress headaches, also known as tension headaches, occur when stress tightens muscles around the scalp, neck, and shoulders, causing pain and discomfort. Migraines can also be triggered or worsened by stress, especially in those with pre-existing susceptibility.
- **Long-Term Effects**: Chronic headaches can lead to fatigue, poor concentration, and irritability, affecting one's quality of life and productivity.
- **Yoga's Role**: Breathing exercises, meditation, and gentle inversions in yoga improve circulation and release physical

and mental tension, often alleviating the intensity and frequency of stress-induced headaches.

3. Digestive Issues

- **How It Manifests**: Stress can disrupt digestion by influencing the gut-brain connection. Common symptoms include stomach aches, bloating, constipation, and irritable bowel syndrome (IBS).
- **Long-Term Effects**: Chronic digestive issues can weaken the gut lining, reduce nutrient absorption, and negatively impact the immune system, as the gut plays a key role in immune health.
- **Yoga's Role**: Gentle twists, forward folds, and deep belly breathing stimulate digestion, calm the nervous system, and help relieve gastrointestinal discomfort.

4. Sleep Disturbances and Fatigue

- **How It Manifests**: Chronic stress affects sleep quality and duration, often resulting in insomnia or light, unrefreshing sleep. Lack of sleep further exacerbates stress, creating a cycle of fatigue and irritability.
- **Long-Term Effects**: Poor sleep weakens the immune system, reduces cognitive function, and impairs mood, making it harder to manage stress effectively.
- **Yoga's Role**: Evening practices focusing on deep relaxation, gentle stretches, and

breathing techniques help ease the body into restful sleep by calming the nervous system.

Tools for Identifying and Addressing Sources of Stress in Daily Life

Managing stress begins with recognizing its sources and understanding how it affects your mind and body. Here are some tools to help you identify and address stress, fostering a healthier relationship with daily challenges.

1. Self-Awareness and Reflection

- **Practice Journaling**: Writing in a journal about your daily experiences can help you identify stress patterns, such as recurring thoughts, emotions, or triggers. Regular reflection also allows you to observe how stress affects your body and mind.
- **Body Scanning**: Body scanning involves mentally checking in with different parts of your body to observe areas of tension or discomfort. This exercise can be part of your yoga practice or done anytime throughout the day, helping you notice and release stress.

2. Set Boundaries and Prioritize Self-Care

- **Define Boundaries**: Set boundaries with work, social obligations, and personal expectations to prevent overcommitment and burnout. Learn to say "no" when needed and give yourself permission to prioritize rest.
- **Schedule Self-Care**: Incorporate self-care activities into your daily or weekly routine. These might include a relaxing yoga session, reading, meditation, or spending time outdoors. Regular self-care builds resilience against stress.

3. Create a Stress Management Plan

- **Identify Triggers**: Make a list of common stressors, such as work deadlines, family obligations, or health concerns. Once identified, you can address these sources of stress proactively, whether by organizing your time, asking for help, or adjusting your mindset.
- **Develop Coping Strategies**: Practice healthy coping strategies, such as deep breathing, mindfulness, or engaging in hobbies you enjoy. These techniques provide quick and effective ways to manage stress as it arises.

4. Build a Support Network

- **Connect with Loved Ones**: Share your thoughts and feelings with trusted friends or family members. Talking through stress can relieve emotional tension, provide perspective, and help you feel less alone.
- **Seek Professional Support**: A therapist, counselor, or yoga instructor specializing in stress relief can offer guidance and additional tools to help you manage chronic stress effectively.

5. Practice Mindful Breathing Techniques

- **Benefits of Breathwork**: Deep, mindful breathing engages the body's relaxation response, slowing the heart rate, reducing blood pressure, and calming the nervous system.
- **Techniques for Stress Relief**: Techniques like diaphragmatic breathing, alternate nostril breathing (Nadi Shodhana), or the 4-7-8 breath can quickly reduce stress and restore a sense of calm. Practicing these techniques throughout your day or during your yoga routine can help you manage stress effectively.

- **Reflection**: Journal about your experiences and observations related to stress in your body. Which physical symptoms have you noticed, and how have they affected your daily life? Reflect on any stressors you identified and note one or two tools you're interested in trying to manage them.

Understanding how stress affects your body and using tools to identify and address its sources can help you make positive changes. Yoga's restorative poses, breathwork, and mindfulness practices will support your journey to relief, equipping you with a foundation for lasting stress management.

Chapter 5: Poses to Release Tension

Overview

In this chapter, we'll explore restorative poses specifically chosen to alleviate physical tension in areas where stress commonly accumulates—namely the neck, shoulders, hips, and back. These poses focus on deep stretching and relaxation, helping to unwind tight muscles and restore a sense of calm. With an emphasis on mindfulness, each pose invites you to relax deeply, letting go of physical and mental tension.

Restorative Poses to Alleviate Tension in Common Stress-Holding Areas

Stress manifests physically by tightening and tensing specific muscles, particularly in the neck, shoulders, hips, and back. Practicing restorative poses can relieve tightness, increase circulation, and promote flexibility, providing both immediate relief and long-term benefits. Here are some of the most effective restorative poses to target these areas.

1. Forward Fold (Uttanasana)

- **Benefits**: Forward Fold stretches the hamstrings, releases tension in the spine, and gently lengthens the back, neck, and shoulders. By inverting the upper body, it also promotes relaxation and circulation.

- **How to Practice**: Stand with your feet hip-width apart. Slowly hinge at the hips, folding your torso forward and allowing your arms to dangle or clasping opposite elbows. Keep a slight bend in your knees if needed to avoid straining your hamstrings. Let your head and neck relax, allowing gravity to create a gentle stretch along your spine.
- **Modifications**: If you feel tight, place your hands on a block for support. You can also bend your knees more deeply for a gentler stretch.

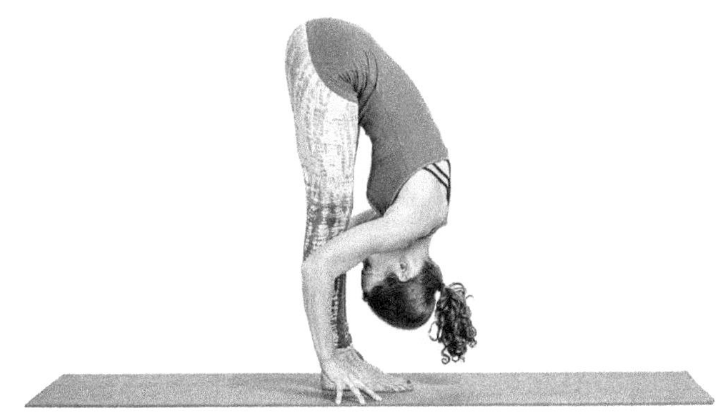

2. Reclined Butterfly (Supta Baddha Konasana)

- **Benefits**: Reclined Butterfly opens the hips and gently stretches the inner thighs and groin. It also promotes deep relaxation, making it an ideal pose for calming both the body and mind.

- **How to Practice**: Lie on your back, bringing the soles of your feet together and allowing your knees to gently fall open, creating a diamond shape with your legs. Place a pillow or blocks under each knee if needed for support. Rest your arms by your sides or place them on your abdomen.
- **Modifications**: If the pose feels too intense on your hips, try placing a pillow or bolster under each knee for added support. You can also place a pillow under your head and neck for added comfort.

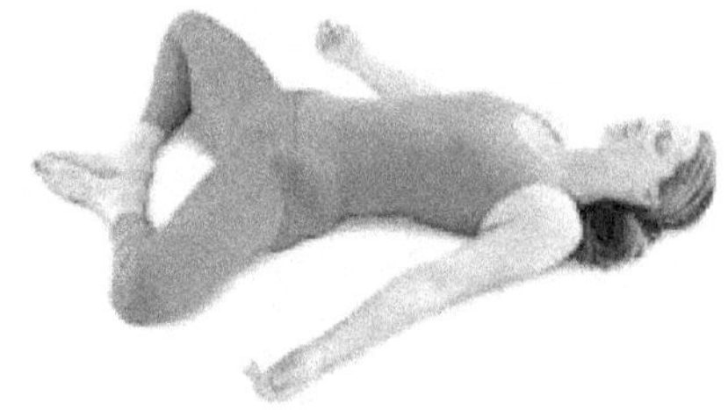

3. Legs-Up-the-Wall (Viparita Karani)

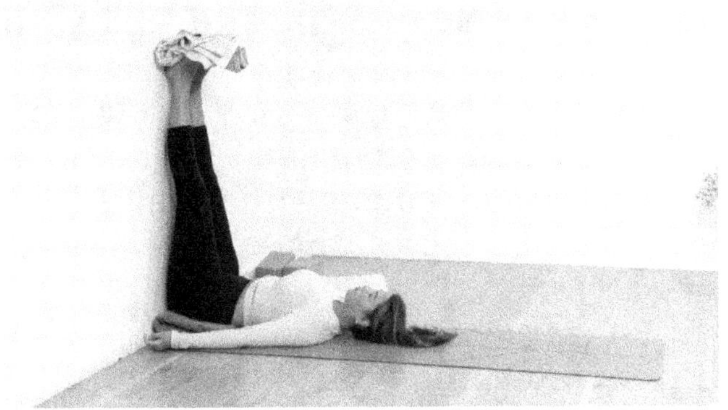

- **Benefits**: This pose helps drain tension from the legs and lower back, reduces swelling, and gently stretches the hamstrings. By inverting the body, it also promotes relaxation and circulation, making it an effective pose for calming the nervous system.
- **How to Practice**: Sit close to a wall, then lie back and extend your legs up the wall, positioning your hips close to the base. Allow your arms to rest by your sides or place one hand on your heart and the other on your abdomen to deepen the connection with your breath.
- **Modifications**: For more support, place a folded blanket or bolster under your hips. If you're uncomfortable with your legs fully extended, try bending your knees slightly or placing a pillow between your legs and the wall.

Focus on Deep Stretching and Relaxation

These poses encourage deep stretching and muscle relaxation, helping release tension on a physical level and quieting the mind. Here are some additional poses that target key stress-holding areas:

4. Supported Child's Pose (Balasana)

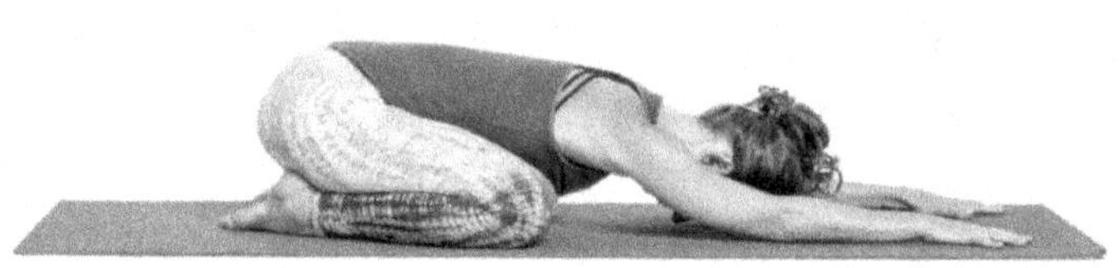

- **Benefits**: Child's Pose stretches the back, shoulders, and hips, providing a soothing release. It's a grounding posture that helps calm the mind and relieve tension.
- **How to Practice**: Kneel on the mat with your big toes touching and knees spread wide. Sit back on your heels and stretch your arms forward, resting your forehead on the mat or a block. You can also rest your chest on a bolster for added support.

- **Modifications**: If you need additional support, place a pillow or bolster under your torso, or keep your knees closer together for a gentler stretch in the lower back.

5.   Cat-Cow   Stretch   (Marjaryasana-Bitilasana)

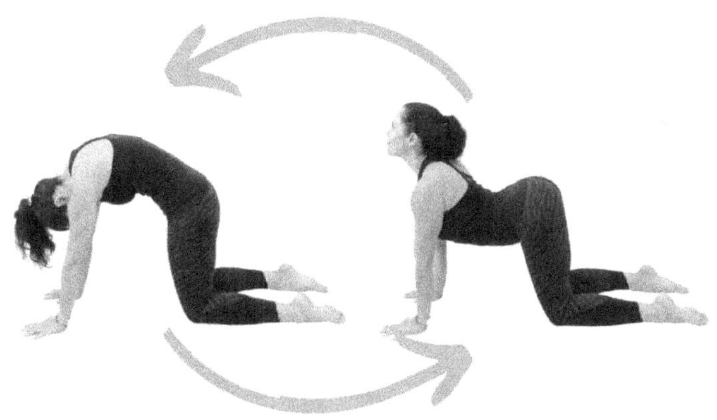

- **Benefits**: This flowing movement between Cat and Cow poses stretches the spine, relieves tension in the back and neck, and helps increase circulation in these areas.
- **How to Practice**: Start on your hands and knees with your wrists directly under your shoulders and knees under your hips. As you inhale, drop your belly, lift your chest, and look forward (Cow Pose). Exhale and round your spine, tucking your chin to your chest (Cat Pose). Continue moving with your breath for several cycles.

- **Modifications**: If your wrists feel strained, place a folded towel under your hands or practice on your forearms.

6. Sphinx Pose (Salamba Bhujangasana)

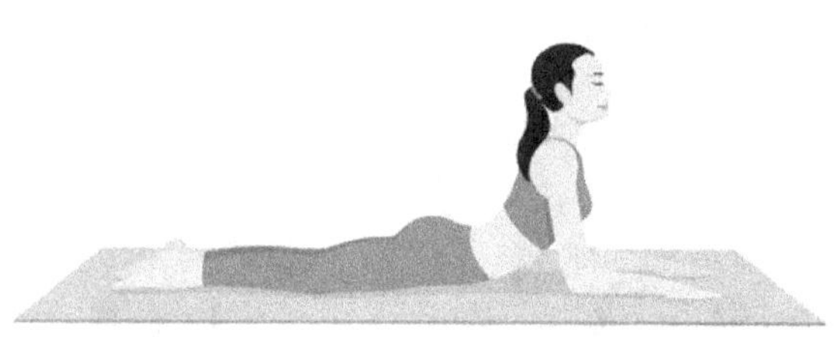

- **Benefits**: Sphinx Pose gently opens the chest, stretches the lower back, and relieves stress-related tension. It's an accessible backbend that promotes a calm, alert state.
- **How to Practice**: Lie on your stomach with your legs extended and elbows under your shoulders. Press your forearms into the mat, lifting your chest while keeping your shoulders relaxed. Hold for several breaths, focusing on lengthening the spine.
- **Modifications**: If you feel tension in your lower back, place a folded blanket under your hips for added support. Avoid lifting too high if it causes discomfort.

Combining Deep Stretching with Mindfulness

As you practice these poses, focus on breathing deeply, using each exhale to release more tension from your body. Here's how to incorporate mindfulness for a more restorative experience:

1. **Slow, Deep Breaths**: Inhale deeply through your nose, filling your lungs completely, and exhale slowly, allowing your body to soften with each breath.
2. **Scan for Tension**: As you move into each pose, perform a quick mental scan of your body to identify any areas of residual tension. Let each exhale help release these areas.
3. **Hold Poses for Extended Periods**: Restorative poses are most effective when held for at least 3-5 minutes. Use props to ensure comfort, and allow your body to ease into the stretch naturally.
4. **Set an Intention for Relaxation**: Remind yourself that this practice is for your healing and restoration. If your mind wanders, bring it back to your breath and the gentle sensations of your body.

Reflection: After practicing these poses, take a few moments to reflect on how your body feels. What changes do you notice in areas of tension like your neck, shoulders, or hips? This awareness will help reinforce the benefits of releasing tension through restorative poses.

By practicing these poses regularly, you'll cultivate greater awareness of stress in your body and learn how to manage it through gentle, mindful movements.

Chapter 6: The Power of Breath in Stress Relief

Overview

The breath is a powerful tool for managing stress, supporting relaxation, and rebalancing the body and mind. In this chapter, we'll explore breathing techniques that activate the body's relaxation response, helping to reduce stress levels and increase mental clarity. Techniques like the 4-7-8 breath, alternate nostril breathing, and breath retention are accessible, effective practices that can be used anytime you feel overwhelmed or need to ground yourself. This chapter provides guided exercises to help you learn and integrate each technique.

Techniques for Stress Relief Through Breath

Breathwork taps into the nervous system, helping to shift the body from a state of stress (sympathetic nervous system activation) to a state of rest and restoration (parasympathetic nervous system activation). Practicing these techniques can reduce stress, improve focus, and promote emotional balance.

1. 4-7-8 Breath

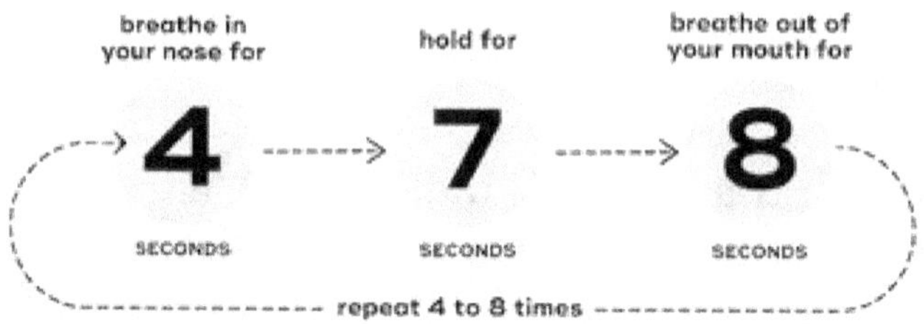

The 4-7-8 breath technique, developed by Dr. Andrew Weil, is designed to promote relaxation by slowing the breath and lengthening exhalation. This practice is especially helpful for calming the mind and relieving stress.

- **How to Practice**:
    1. Sit comfortably with your back straight, either on a chair or on the floor.
    2. Place the tip of your tongue against the roof of your mouth, just behind your front teeth.
    3. Inhale quietly through your nose to a count of 4.
    4. Hold your breath for a count of 7.
    5. Exhale completely through your mouth, making a "whooshing" sound, for a count of 8.
    6. Repeat the cycle for four breaths to start, gradually working up to eight cycles as you build comfort with the practice.

- **Benefits**: The 4-7-8 breath relaxes the nervous system, improves focus, and promotes a sense of calm. It's particularly effective for easing anxiety or helping to unwind before sleep.

2. Alternate Nostril Breathing (Nadi Shodhana)

Alternate nostril breathing, or Nadi Shodhana, is a technique that balances energy and calms the mind. By breathing through each nostril individually, this practice harmonizes the two hemispheres of the brain, improving focus and reducing stress.

- **How to Practice**:
    1. Sit comfortably with your spine straight and shoulders relaxed.
    2. Place your right thumb on your right nostril and your ring finger on your left nostril.
    3. Close your right nostril with your thumb and inhale slowly through the left nostril.
    4. Close the left nostril with your ring finger and release your thumb from the right nostril, exhaling slowly through the right.
    5. Inhale through the right nostril, then close it with your thumb, and exhale through the left.
    6. This completes one round. Repeat for 5-10 rounds, or about 5 minutes.

- **Benefits**: This practice is excellent for mental clarity, balancing energy, and calming the nervous system. It helps alleviate stress, improves focus, and can support mental clarity during times of overwhelm.

3. Breath Retention (Kumbhaka)

Breath retention, or Kumbhaka, involves holding the breath at certain intervals within the breathing cycle. When practiced mindfully, it builds lung capacity, strengthens the diaphragm, and promotes calmness by briefly increasing oxygen in the blood.

- **How to Practice**:
    1. Begin by inhaling slowly through the nose for a count of 4.
    2. Retain the breath at the top of the inhalation for a comfortable length (aim for a count of 4 to start).
    3. Exhale slowly through the nose for a count of 4.
    4. Rest for a few normal breaths before beginning again, practicing 3-5 cycles in total.
    5. Over time, you may increase the duration of breath retention, but start with short, manageable counts to avoid dizziness.
- **Benefits**: Kumbhaka reduces anxiety, increases breath control, and brings a sense of calm and focus. It strengthens the

respiratory system and promotes mental clarity, making it effective for stress relief.

Guided Exercises to Practice These Techniques

Each of these breathing techniques is most effective when practiced regularly. Below are guided exercises to help you integrate these techniques into your daily routine.

Exercise 1: Morning Breath Practice with 4-7-8 Breath

- **Goal**: Begin your day with clarity and calmness by practicing the 4-7-8 breath.
- **Instructions**: Find a quiet space to sit comfortably. Practice the 4-7-8 breath for five cycles, taking a short rest between each one if needed. Focus on filling your lungs completely on each inhale and releasing all tension on each exhale.
- **Duration**: 5 minutes.

Exercise 2: Midday Stress Relief with Alternate Nostril Breathing

- **Goal**: Relieve midday stress and reset your energy levels by practicing alternate nostril breathing.
- **Instructions**: Sit in a comfortable, upright position and place one hand on your

nostrils to guide your breath. Practice 5-10 rounds, focusing on smooth, even breaths. Feel the calming effect as you balance each inhale and exhale.

- **Duration**: 5 minutes.

Exercise 3: Evening Wind-Down with Breath Retention

- **Goal**: Ease into a relaxed state before sleep by practicing breath retention.
- **Instructions**: Lie down in a comfortable position. Practice the Kumbhaka breath retention, inhaling for a count of 4, holding for a count of 4, and exhaling for a count of 4. Repeat for 3-5 cycles.
- **Duration**: 5-10 minutes.

Benefits of Incorporating Breathwork into Your Daily Routine

1. **Reduces Stress and Anxiety**: Breathing exercises lower cortisol levels, slowing the body's stress response.
2. **Improves Focus and Concentration**: By balancing oxygen and blood flow, these practices increase mental clarity and focus.
3. **Enhances Sleep Quality**: Techniques like the 4-7-8 breath prepare the body for restful sleep by calming the nervous system.

4. **Boosts Lung Capacity and Circulation**: Deep, controlled breathing strengthens the lungs, improves circulation, and increases energy.

Breathwork is a versatile tool for immediate and cumulative stress relief. Integrating these techniques into your routine can transform how you handle stress, supporting greater calmness, clarity, and resilience in all areas of life.

Week 3: Managing Pain with Targeted Yoga Practices

Goal: Focus on poses and routines for pain relief in specific areas like the back, shoulders, and hips.

Chapter 7: Yoga for Back Pain Relief

Overview

Back pain is one of the most common physical complaints, affecting people of all ages and lifestyles. Causes can range from muscle strain to poor posture, stress, or even sitting for long periods. Yoga can be an effective tool for relieving back pain, as it gently strengthens the muscles around the spine, increases flexibility, and encourages relaxation. This chapter explores some of the root causes of back pain and introduces a series of poses designed to target and alleviate tension in the back.

Understanding the Causes of Back Pain and How Yoga Can Help

Back pain can arise from various sources:

- **Poor Posture**: Slouching, hunching over a desk, or tilting the head forward for prolonged periods creates stress on the spine.
- **Muscle Imbalance**: Weak or tight muscles in the lower back, hips, and abdomen can cause misalignment, leading to back discomfort.
- **Stress and Tension**: Stress often manifests in physical tension, particularly in the neck, shoulders, and lower back.

- **Inactivity or Overuse**: A sedentary lifestyle or sudden intense activity can contribute to back strain and stiffness.

Yoga helps by promoting muscle balance, improving posture, and gently releasing tension. Through mindful movement, you can strengthen and lengthen the back muscles, providing relief from pain and helping to prevent future issues.

Poses and Sequences for Back Pain Relief

The following poses focus on improving flexibility, reducing tension, and strengthening key muscles to alleviate back pain. Practice each pose slowly and mindfully, listening to your body and adjusting as needed.

1. Cat-Cow Pose (Marjaryasana-Bitilasana)

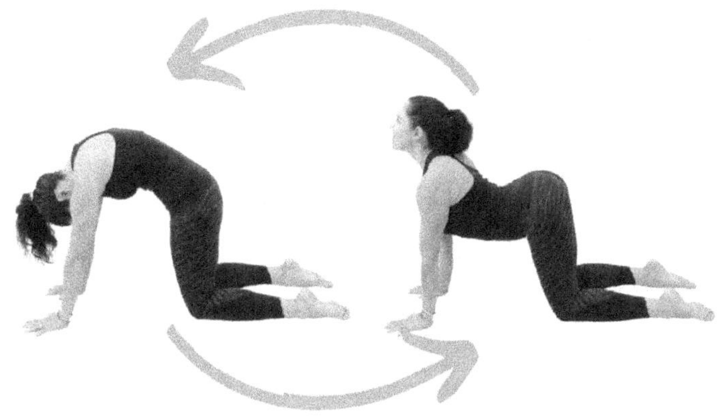

- **Benefits**: This gentle flowing sequence stretches the entire spine, improves circulation to the back, and releases tension in the lower back and shoulders.
- **How to Practice**:
    1. Start on all fours with your wrists aligned under your shoulders and knees under your hips.
    2. On an inhale, drop your belly, lift your chest, and look forward to create a gentle arch in your back (Cow Pose).
    3. Exhale as you round your spine, tucking your chin to your chest and drawing your navel toward your spine (Cat Pose).
    4. Continue to alternate between Cat and Cow poses for 5-10 rounds, linking each movement with your breath.

2. Cobra Pose (Bhujangasana)

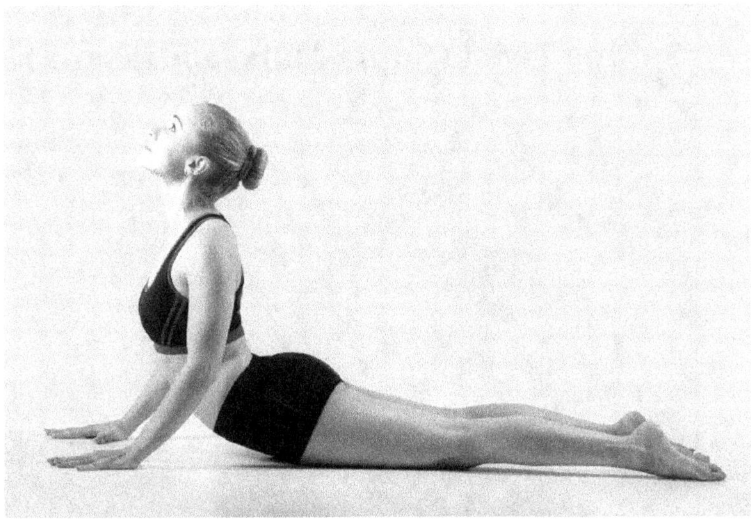

- **Benefits**: Cobra Pose strengthens the back muscles, stretches the chest, and improves flexibility in the spine, helping to counteract the effects of poor posture.
- **How to Practice**:
    1. Lie on your stomach with your legs extended and your palms on the floor under your shoulders.
    2. Press through your hands to lift your chest, keeping your elbows slightly bent and close to your body.
    3. Gaze forward or slightly upward, extending through the crown of your head.
    4. Hold for a few breaths, focusing on lengthening your spine as you lift.
- **Modifications**: If the pose feels too intense, lower halfway or place your

forearms on the mat (Sphinx Pose) for a gentler backbend.

3. Supine Twist (Supta Matsyendrasana)

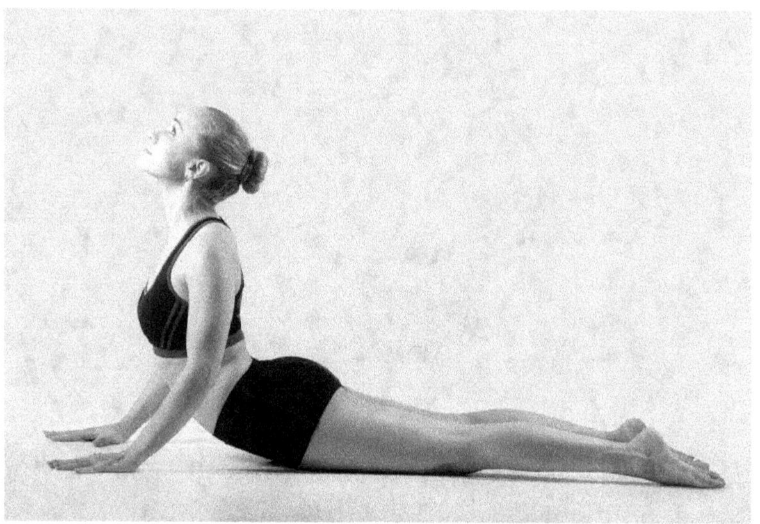

- **Benefits**: This reclining twist relieves tension in the lower back, massages the spine, and helps to release tight muscles along the back and hips.
- **How to Practice**:
    1. Lie on your back with your knees bent and feet flat on the floor.
    2. Draw your right knee to your chest and extend your left leg on the floor.
    3. Gently guide your right knee across your body to the left, reaching your right arm out to the side.
    4. Keep both shoulders grounded as you twist, holding for several breaths.
    5. Repeat on the opposite side.

Creating a Routine for Back Pain Relief

Combining these poses into a sequence allows you to address back tension comprehensively:

1. **Begin with Cat-Cow** to warm up the spine, moving fluidly for 5-10 rounds.
2. **Move to Cobra Pose**, holding for 3-5 breaths to strengthen the back and open the chest.
3. **Finish with Supine Twist** on each side, holding for at least 5 breaths to release any residual tension.

Repeat this routine daily, or as often as needed, to manage back discomfort and gradually improve flexibility and strength in the spine.

Tips for Practicing Yoga for Back Pain Relief

1. **Consistency is Key**: Practicing these poses regularly is more effective than occasional long sessions. Aim for short daily routines to see lasting improvement.
2. **Focus on Breath**: Use your breath to enhance relaxation and release tension, especially in poses that feel intense.
3. **Listen to Your Body**: Back pain varies, so honor your body's limits and avoid any movements that worsen your discomfort.

4. **Strengthen Supporting Muscles**:
Include poses that strengthen the core,
hips, and legs to support spinal health and
prevent back pain.

This chapter emphasizes mindful movement,
breathing, and gentle stretches to alleviate back
pain. By incorporating these poses into your
routine, you can nurture a strong, flexible spine
and experience long-term relief from back
tension.

Chapter 8: Yoga for Neck and Shoulder Pain

Overview

Neck and shoulder pain are common, often due to stress, poor posture, and sedentary habits like prolonged desk work. Yoga offers gentle, effective ways to release this tension, restoring flexibility and balance. In this chapter, we'll explore some of the main causes of neck and shoulder pain and introduce poses that target these areas, such as Eagle Arms, Shoulder Rolls, and Neck Stretches, to alleviate discomfort and improve mobility.

Understanding the Causes of Neck and Shoulder Pain

Several factors contribute to neck and shoulder pain, including:

- **Poor Posture**: Slouching, craning the neck forward, or rounding the shoulders puts strain on the neck and upper back muscles.
- **Stress and Tension**: Stress often manifests physically, leading to muscle tightness, particularly in the shoulders, neck, and jaw.
- **Sedentary Lifestyle**: Spending extended periods sitting, especially with minimal movement, can lead to muscle imbalances

and restricted movement in the upper body.

Yoga helps alleviate this pain by gently stretching and strengthening the muscles around the neck and shoulders, improving posture, and encouraging relaxation.

Poses to Alleviate Neck and Shoulder Pain

The following yoga poses target tension in the neck and shoulders, helping to release stress and restore natural mobility. Practice each pose slowly and mindfully, focusing on deep breathing to enhance relaxation.

1. Eagle Arms (Garudasana Arms)

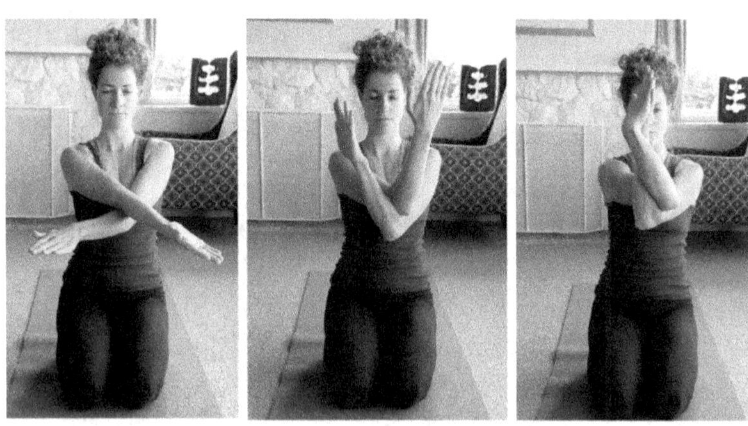

- **Benefits**: This pose opens the shoulder blades and stretches the upper back, releasing tension in the shoulders and neck.

- **How to Practice**:
  1. Sit or stand comfortably with a straight spine.
  2. Extend your arms forward at shoulder height and cross your right arm over your left, bringing your palms together or grabbing opposite shoulders if your palms don't touch.
  3. Lift your elbows slightly and press your forearms forward to deepen the stretch.
  4. Hold for several breaths, then switch sides.

2. Shoulder Rolls

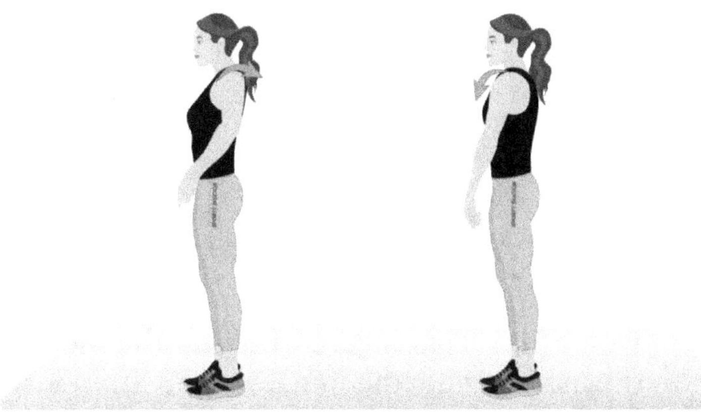

- **Benefits**: Shoulder rolls are a simple yet effective way to release tightness and improve circulation in the shoulder joints and neck.
- **How to Practice**:

1. Sit or stand with your arms relaxed at your sides.
2. Inhale as you lift your shoulders up toward your ears, then roll them back and down on an exhale.
3. Repeat for 5-10 rounds, then switch directions, rolling your shoulders forward.

3. Neck Stretch

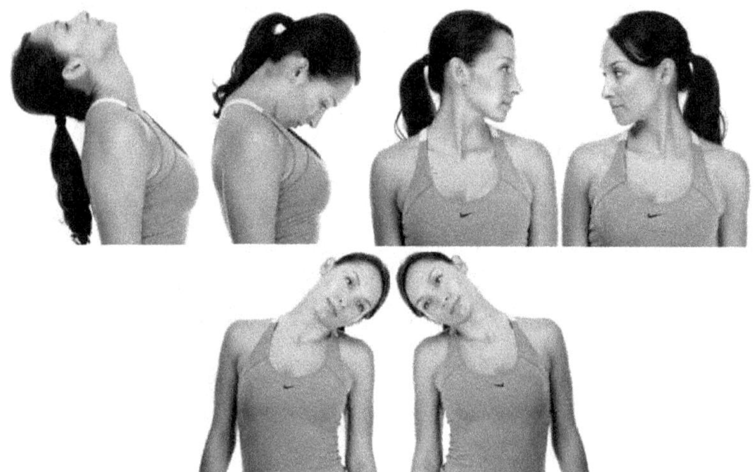

- **Benefits**: This stretch targets the sides of the neck, relieving tension and improving flexibility.
- **How to Practice**:
    1. Sit comfortably with your spine tall.
    2. Gently tilt your head to the right, bringing your right ear toward your right shoulder.

3. For a deeper stretch, place your right hand on the left side of your head and apply gentle pressure.
4. Hold for a few breaths, then switch sides.

Creating a Routine for Neck and Shoulder Pain Relief

These poses can be easily integrated into a short routine:

1. **Begin with Shoulder Rolls** to warm up the shoulders and neck, moving in both directions for 10-15 rounds.
2. **Move into Eagle Arms** on each side, holding for 5-10 breaths to open up the upper back and shoulder blades.
3. **Finish with the Neck Stretch** on both sides, holding each stretch for 5-10 breaths to release tension in the sides of the neck.

Practicing this routine regularly, especially after long periods of sitting, can prevent tension from building up in the neck and shoulders.

Tips for Practicing Yoga for Neck and Shoulder Pain Relief

1. **Practice Regularly**: Short, consistent practice is more effective than occasional

long sessions, especially when managing neck and shoulder tension.

2. **Use Deep Breathing**: Breathwork helps reduce tension and promotes relaxation, making stretches more effective.

3. **Move Slowly and Mindfully**: Avoid sudden movements, which can increase neck strain. Move gently and stay aware of your limits.

This chapter offers gentle poses and mindful movements to relieve neck and shoulder pain. By practicing these regularly, you can improve mobility, reduce pain, and prevent future tension in these common stress-holding areas.

Chapter 9: Yoga for Hip Pain and Sciatica Relief

Overview

Hip pain and sciatica are common issues that can significantly affect daily activities and overall quality of life. Hip tension often stems from prolonged sitting, lack of mobility, and stress, while sciatica—a type of nerve pain that radiates along the sciatic nerve from the lower back down through the hips and legs—can be caused by muscle imbalances or tightness around the hip joint. In this chapter, we'll explore how yoga can help relieve these issues through hip-opening poses, focusing on releasing tight muscles, improving mobility, and easing sciatic discomfort.

Understanding Hip Tension and Sciatica

- **Hip Tension**: The hips are a major intersection in the body, carrying the weight of the upper body and connecting it to the lower body. Prolonged sitting, lack of movement, and even emotional stress can contribute to tightness in the hip area, particularly in the hip flexors and glutes. This tension can lead to discomfort or pain in the hips, lower back, and legs.
- **Sciatica**: Sciatic pain occurs when the sciatic nerve, which runs from the lower spine down each leg, becomes irritated or

compressed. Tightness in the hip muscles, especially the piriformis muscle, can aggravate the sciatic nerve, resulting in pain that radiates down the leg.

Yoga's focus on hip-opening poses helps by loosening tight muscles, increasing blood flow to the area, and relieving pressure on the sciatic nerve, which in turn helps to alleviate pain and restore mobility.

Poses for Hip Pain and Sciatica Relief

The following poses target tight hip muscles and help release tension along the sciatic nerve pathway. Practice each pose slowly, using your breath to guide you into deeper stretches.

1. Pigeon Pose (Eka Pada Rajakapotasana)

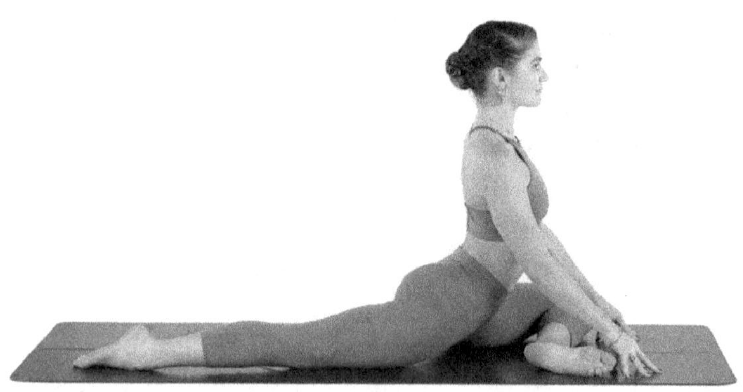

- **Benefits**: Pigeon Pose is one of the most effective hip openers, stretching the hip flexors, glutes, and piriformis muscle. It can relieve tension that aggravates sciatica.
- **How to Practice**:
    1. Start in a tabletop position and bring your right knee forward, placing it behind your right wrist.
    2. Extend your left leg straight back, keeping your hips square.
    3. Lower your torso forward over your right shin, resting on your forearms or forehead.
    4. Hold for several breaths, then switch sides.
- **Modifications**: Place a cushion under the hip or lower leg for support if this stretch is too intense.

2. Reclined Figure Four (Supta Kapotasana)

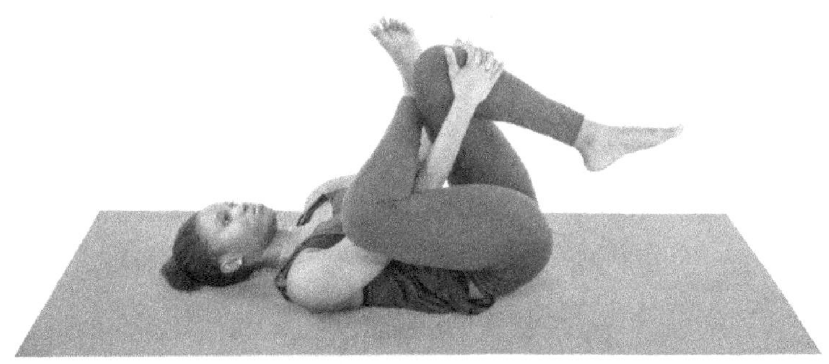

- **Benefits**: Reclined Figure Four gently opens the hips and stretches the piriformis muscle, providing relief from sciatic pain.
- **How to Practice**:
    1. Lie on your back with both knees bent and feet flat on the floor.
    2. Cross your right ankle over your left thigh, creating a "4" shape.
    3. Draw your left thigh toward you, threading your arms through to clasp behind the thigh or knee.
    4. Hold for several breaths, then switch sides.

3. Low Lunge (Anjaneyasana)

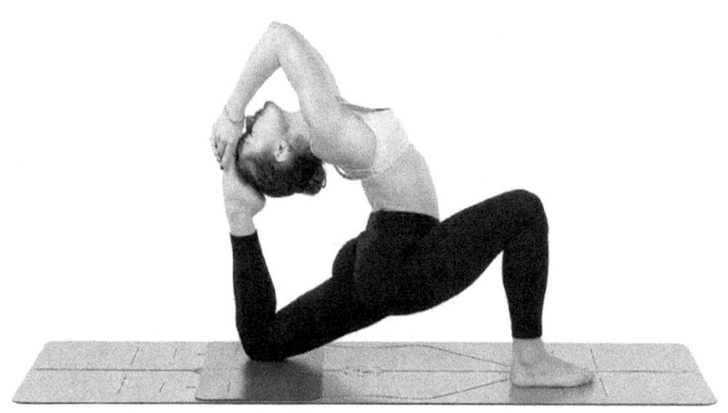

- **Benefits**: Low Lunge stretches the hip flexors and quadriceps, helping to release tension and increase flexibility in the hips.
- **How to Practice**:
    1. From a tabletop position, step your right foot forward between your

hands, aligning your knee over your ankle.
2. Lower your left knee to the floor and lift your torso upright, placing your hands on your front thigh or reaching them overhead.
3. Hold for several breaths, feeling the stretch in your left hip, then switch sides.

- **Modifications**: Place a blanket or cushion under your back knee for extra support.

Creating a Routine for Hip Pain and Sciatica Relief

This routine combines the above poses to provide targeted relief for hip pain and sciatica. Move through the poses mindfully, allowing each stretch to release tension gradually.

1. **Start with Low Lunge** on each side, holding for 5-10 breaths to warm up the hip flexors and quadriceps.
2. **Move into Reclined Figure Four** on each side, holding for 5-10 breaths to gently release the glutes and piriformis.
3. **Finish with Pigeon Pose** on each side, holding for 5-10 breaths to deeply open the hips and relieve sciatic tension.

Practicing this sequence regularly can help reduce hip pain and ease sciatic discomfort, allowing for improved mobility and overall comfort.

Tips for Practicing Yoga for Hip Pain and Sciatica Relief

1. **Use Props for Support**: Blankets or blocks can help make these poses more accessible and comfortable, especially if your hips are tight.
2. **Move Slowly**: Avoid pushing too hard, especially in deep hip openers. Allow the muscles to gradually release with each breath.
3. **Focus on Breath**: Deep breathing helps relax the muscles around the hips, allowing for a deeper, more effective stretch.

This chapter provides targeted poses and mindful movements to relieve hip pain and sciatica. By incorporating these poses into your routine, you can gradually reduce tension, improve flexibility, and experience lasting relief in the hips and lower back.

Week 4: Boosting Energy and Combating Fatigue

Goal: Use energizing sequences and mindfulness techniques to boost energy and combat chronic fatigue.

Chapter 10: The Role of Energy in Yoga

Overview

In yoga, energy is a vital concept, often referred to as prana, or life energy. Prana is believed to be the essential force that flows through the body, supporting physical and mental well-being. When energy flows freely, we feel balanced, revitalized, and grounded. However, energy "leaks" or blockages—due to stress, poor posture, or even negative emotions—can disrupt this flow, leading to fatigue, mental fog, and a sense of imbalance. In this chapter, we'll explore prana, how yoga restores energy flow, and how specific practices can help you replenish energy levels.

Understanding Prana (Life Energy) and How Yoga Restores Energy Flow

- **What is Prana?**: Prana is the vital life force that sustains our physical and mental energy. It flows through energy channels called nadis, which are similar to the concept of meridians in Traditional Chinese

Medicine. When prana flows harmoniously, we experience physical health, mental clarity, and emotional stability.

- **Energy Centers (Chakras)**: Prana is concentrated in seven primary chakras, or energy centers, located along the spine. Each chakra corresponds to specific physical and emotional qualities. Yoga postures, breathing techniques, and meditation help keep these chakras balanced, which ensures a steady flow of prana throughout the body.
- **Restoring Energy Flow with Yoga**: Yoga encourages a free flow of prana by moving the body in ways that open the energy channels, release physical blockages, and calm the mind. Poses that expand the chest, lengthen the spine, and strengthen the core support the movement of prana, while breathing techniques (pranayama) invigorate the body and help clear stagnant energy.

Identifying Energy "Leaks" and How Yoga Helps Replenish Energy Levels

Energy leaks occur when we feel drained, fatigued, or emotionally scattered. They can be caused by:

- **Poor Posture**: Slouching or sitting for prolonged periods compresses the chest and restricts prana flow.
- **Mental and Emotional Stress**: Anxiety, fear, and negative thinking can sap our energy, leaving us feeling depleted.
- **Overcommitment and Exhaustion**: Busy schedules and lack of rest lead to energy imbalances, creating a state of chronic fatigue.

Yoga addresses these leaks by:

- **Improving Posture**: Postures that lengthen the spine, open the chest, and strengthen core muscles help support natural prana flow.
- **Reducing Stress and Calming the Mind**: By connecting breath with movement, yoga helps reduce stress and anxiety, encouraging relaxation and replenishing energy.
- **Encouraging Restorative Practices**: Gentle or restorative yoga poses promote deep relaxation, giving the body time to replenish prana and restore energy balance.

Practices to Replenish Energy Levels

The following yoga practices are particularly helpful in restoring and conserving energy:

1. **Breath of Fire (Kapalabhati)**:
   - **Purpose**: This energizing breathing technique helps clear mental fog, boost energy, and improve focus.
   - **How to Practice**: Sit comfortably, take a deep inhale, then exhale rapidly by contracting your abdomen while keeping the inhale passive. Continue for 1-2 minutes.
2. **Heart-Opening Poses (e.g., Bridge Pose, Camel Pose)**:
   - **Purpose**: These poses expand the chest, allowing for greater oxygen intake and a surge of fresh energy to circulate through the body.
   - **How to Practice**: Hold each pose for several breaths, focusing on inhaling deeply to expand the chest and energize the body.
3. **Savasana (Corpse Pose)**:
   - **Purpose**: Savasana is a deeply restorative pose that allows the body to absorb the benefits of the practice, replenishing prana and grounding energy.
   - **How to Practice**: Lie on your back, arms at your sides, with your palms facing up. Close your eyes and focus on your breath, letting go of tension in each part of your body. Stay for at least 5-10 minutes.

Summary of Chapter 10 Practices

Understanding prana and the role of energy in yoga is fundamental for managing your vitality and well-being. By integrating breathing techniques, energy-restoring poses, and stress-reducing practices into your routine, you can nurture a balanced flow of energy, avoid energy leaks, and experience a renewed sense of mental and physical clarity.

Chapter 11: Morning Yoga Routines for Energy

Overview

Starting the day with a focused and energizing yoga routine can set a positive tone, boosting energy levels and mental clarity for the hours ahead. Morning yoga wakes up the body, enhances circulation, and brings a fresh flow of energy to the mind. In this chapter, we'll explore short morning routines designed to invigorate, including dynamic sequences like Sun Salutations and powerful poses such as Warrior and Tree Pose.

Benefits of Morning Yoga Routines

Practicing yoga in the morning has unique benefits:

- **Improves Alertness and Focus**: Movement and deep breathing help stimulate circulation and oxygenate the body, sharpening focus and concentration.
- **Releases Tension**: Gentle stretching and movement release stiffness from sleep, preparing the body for the demands of the day.
- **Enhances Mood and Positivity**: Starting with mindful movement and deep breathing creates a sense of calm and

positivity, which can carry into your interactions and activities.

Key Poses for Morning Energy

These poses are ideal for activating the body and mind in the morning. Focus on your breath and alignment to experience the full benefit of each movement.

1. Sun Salutations (Surya Namaskar)

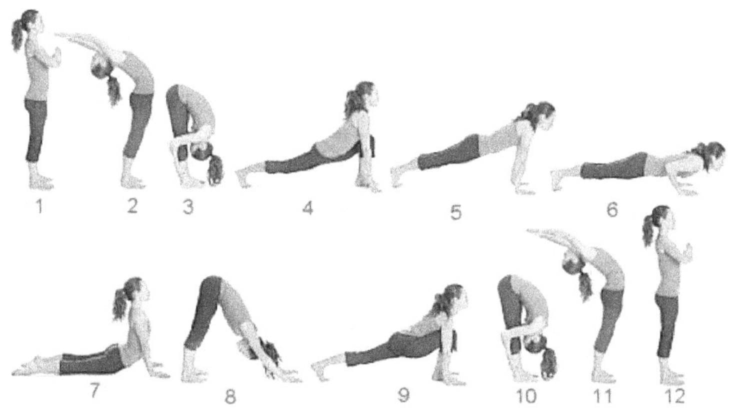

- **Purpose**: Sun Salutations are a traditional, flowing sequence of poses that build heat, improve flexibility, and increase circulation, making them perfect for warming up in the morning.
- **How to Practice**:
    1. Start in Mountain Pose, standing tall with hands at your heart.

2. Inhale as you raise your arms overhead, then exhale as you fold forward.
3. Move through a sequence of poses, including Plank, Cobra, and Downward-Facing Dog, before returning to standing.
4. Repeat 3-5 times for a quick, energizing start.

2. Warrior Pose (Virabhadrasana)

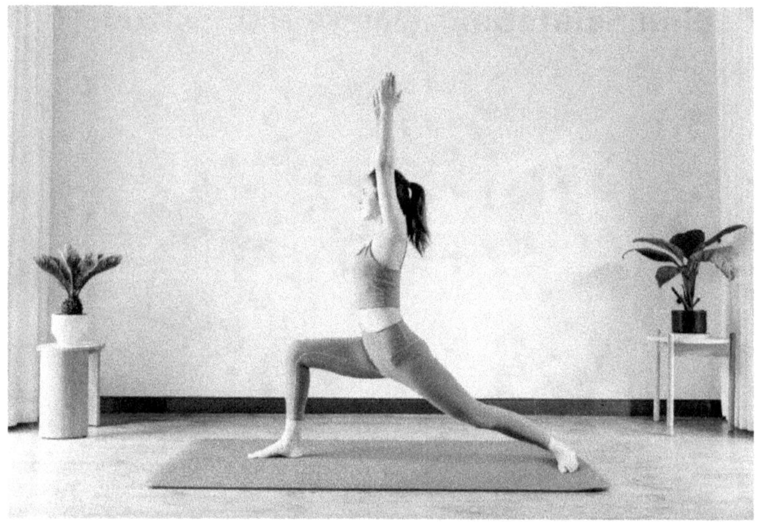

- **Purpose**: Warrior poses build strength, balance, and confidence, awakening the legs and engaging the core for stability.
- **How to Practice**:
    1. Step your right foot back, turning the toes slightly outward, and bend your left knee over the ankle.

2. Raise your arms overhead or extend them parallel to the floor, keeping your gaze forward.
3. Hold for several breaths, then switch sides.

3. Tree Pose (Vrksasana)

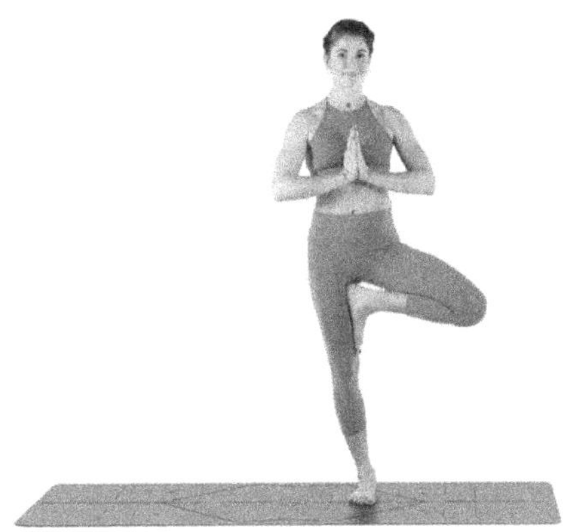

- **Purpose**: This balancing pose enhances mental focus and grounding, preparing you to approach the day with poise and clarity.
- **How to Practice**:
    1. Stand on your left foot, bringing the sole of your right foot to the inside of your left thigh or calf.
    2. Bring your hands together at your chest or raise them overhead.
    3. Focus on a point in front of you for balance, holding for several breaths, then switch sides.

Sample Morning Routine

This routine combines dynamic poses and grounding balances to activate your body and mind:

1. **Begin with 3 Rounds of Sun Salutations** to warm up the muscles and stimulate circulation.
2. **Transition to Warrior Pose** on each side, holding for 3-5 breaths per side to build strength and endurance.
3. **Finish with Tree Pose** on each side, holding for 5 breaths to center yourself and enhance balance.

This short sequence can be done in under 10 minutes, making it easy to integrate into even the busiest mornings.

Tips for Practicing Morning Yoga

1. **Practice on an Empty Stomach**: To avoid discomfort, practice yoga before eating breakfast, or wait 1-2 hours after eating.
2. **Focus on Deep Breathing**: Deep, controlled breaths help wake up the body and improve oxygen flow, making each movement more energizing.
3. **Stay Mindful**: Use this time to check in with your body and mind, setting an intention for the day to carry the positive energy forward.

This chapter provides a practical guide to energizing morning routines. By incorporating Sun Salutations, Warrior, and Tree Pose into your morning, you can cultivate energy, strength, and mental clarity, empowering yourself to start each day on a high note.

Chapter 12: Evening Yoga for Deep Rest and Restoration

Overview

An evening yoga routine offers a gentle way to unwind from the day, preparing the body and mind for restful sleep. Evening yoga focuses on slow, grounding movements, releasing tension, and calming the nervous system, which helps to counteract the day's stress and promote deep relaxation. In this chapter, we'll explore soothing poses and deep breathing exercises that encourage relaxation, including practices like Supine Twist, Happy Baby, and Savasana.

Benefits of Evening Yoga for Rest and Restoration

Practicing yoga before bed can be beneficial in numerous ways:

- **Reduces Muscle Tension**: Gentle stretches relieve tightness accumulated from daily activities and sitting for extended periods.
- **Calms the Nervous System**: Slow, deep breathing and restorative poses activate the parasympathetic nervous system, encouraging a relaxation response.
- **Prepares the Mind for Rest**: By focusing on slow, mindful movements and

deep breathing, evening yoga reduces mental clutter, preparing you for a peaceful night's sleep.

Key Poses for Evening Relaxation

These poses are ideal for slowing down and grounding the body before bed, making it easier to transition into restful sleep.

1. Supine Twist (Supta Matsyendrasana)

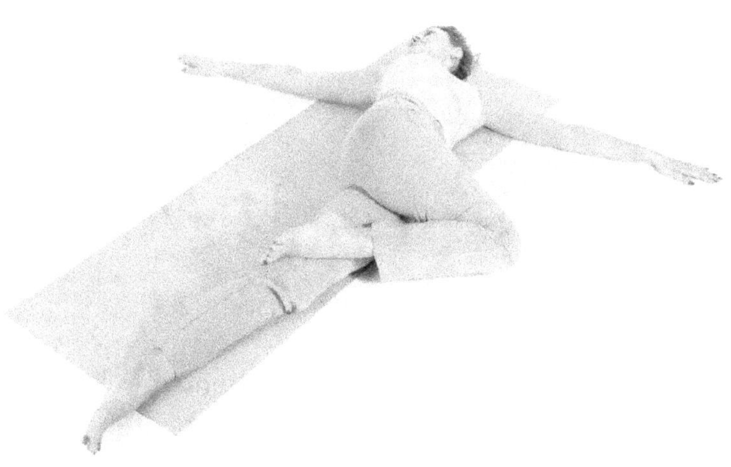

- **Purpose**: This gentle twist releases tension in the spine, hips, and shoulders, easing physical stress and promoting relaxation.
- **How to Practice**:
    1. Lie on your back and bring your knees up to your chest.

2. Lower both knees to the right side, extending your arms out in a "T" shape.
3. Hold for several deep breaths, feeling the gentle stretch through your spine, then switch sides.

2. Happy Baby (Ananda Balasana)

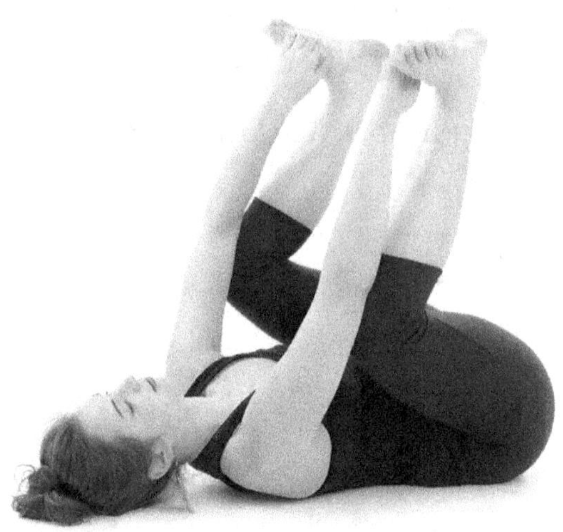

- **Purpose**: Happy Baby pose gently opens the hips, relieves lower back tension, and promotes a sense of grounding and calm.
- **How to Practice**:
    1. Lie on your back, bend your knees, and bring them up toward your chest.
    2. Grab the outer edges of your feet, with your knees wider than your torso.

3. Rock gently side to side for a soothing stretch, holding for several breaths.

3. Savasana (Corpse Pose)

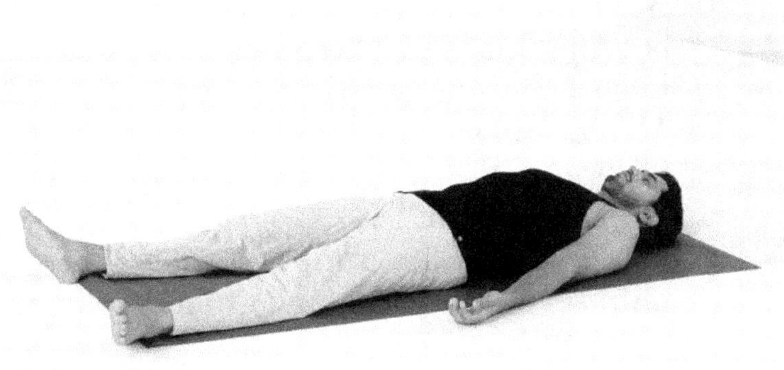

- **Purpose**: Savasana is a deeply relaxing pose that allows the body to absorb the benefits of the practice, transitioning smoothly into rest.
- **How to Practice**:
    1. Lie on your back with arms at your sides, palms facing up.
    2. Close your eyes, focus on slow, deep breathing, and let go of any remaining tension.
    3. Stay for 5-10 minutes, focusing on each part of the body to release any lingering tension.

Sample Evening Routine

This routine is designed to relax the body, release tension, and calm the mind, setting the stage for a peaceful night's sleep.

1. **Begin with Supine Twist** on each side, holding for 5-10 breaths to stretch and release the spine and shoulders.
2. **Move into Happy Baby** to release tension in the lower back and hips, holding for several breaths.
3. **End with Savasana**, staying for 5-10 minutes to fully relax and ground yourself.

Tips for Practicing Evening Yoga

1. **Set a Calming Environment**: Dim the lights, play soft music, or light a candle to create a tranquil space that signals the body to unwind.
2. **Focus on Breath**: Deep, slow breathing helps relax the body and mind, enhancing the calming effects of each pose.
3. **Consistency is Key**: Practicing a short routine each night can condition your body and mind to expect relaxation before bed, making it easier to fall asleep.

Summary of Chapter 12 Practices

This chapter offers evening practices focused on relaxation and restoration. Through gentle poses like Supine Twist, Happy Baby, and Savasana, you can release tension and quiet the mind, supporting a smooth transition from the busyness of the day into a restful, rejuvenating sleep.

Week 5: Integrating the Practice for Long-Term Benefits

Goal: Emphasize sustainability and integrating yoga into daily life to maintain benefits.

Chapter 13: Reflecting on the Journey

Overview

As you reach the end of this 30-day journey with yoga, it's essential to pause, reflect, and appreciate the progress you've made. Reflection allows us to recognize the changes, challenges, and successes experienced along the way. In this chapter, we'll use guided journaling prompts to explore the impact of yoga on your mental and physical health, deepen your awareness, and encourage future growth.

The Importance of Reflection in Personal Growth

Reflecting on a new journey, especially one as transformative as a month of consistent yoga practice, offers multiple benefits:

- **Reinforces Positive Change**: Reflection helps solidify the new habits and perspectives you've developed, increasing the likelihood of long-term growth.

- **Builds Self-Awareness**: Through introspection, you gain a deeper understanding of how yoga has influenced your body, mind, and overall well-being.
- **Encourages Future Commitment**: Acknowledging your successes and challenges motivates you to continue practicing and maintaining the benefits you've achieved.

Journaling Prompts for Reflection

Consider setting aside time to journal, reflecting honestly on the journey and capturing your thoughts on paper. Use these prompts to guide your reflections:

1. **Changes in Physical Health**:
   - How has yoga impacted your strength, flexibility, and overall physical health?
   - Are there specific areas of tension or pain that have lessened since you began?
2. **Mental and Emotional Shifts**:
   - What changes have you noticed in your mood, mindset, or stress levels?
   - How has practicing yoga influenced your emotional resilience?
3. **Challenges and Insights**:

o What challenges did you face along the way, and how did you work through them?
   o Were there any surprising insights or "aha" moments during your practice?
4. **Successes and Achievements**:
   o What aspects of your yoga journey are you most proud of?
   o How has your confidence or self-perception evolved over the past 30 days?
5. **Moving Forward**:
   o Which practices or routines resonated most with you, and how might you incorporate them into your daily life?
   o What are your intentions or goals for your ongoing yoga practice?

Reflecting on Physical and Mental Health

After 30 days of dedicated yoga practice, many people experience a variety of changes in both physical and mental health:

- **Physical Health**: Increased flexibility, improved strength, reduced pain, and better posture are common physical benefits.
- **Mental Health**: Many practitioners report feeling more centered, less stressed, and more present in their daily lives.

By documenting these changes, you can capture the full extent of yoga's impact on your well-being, making it easier to stay motivated and carry forward the benefits.

This final chapter is about taking the time to reflect and celebrate your growth. Through journaling, you can appreciate your progress, reinforce the positive changes, and set intentions for the future. Remember, this journey doesn't end here—your practice is something you can carry forward, evolving along with you as you continue to explore the transformative power of yoga.

Chapter 14: Creating a Personalized Practice

Overview

Now that you've completed 30 days of guided practice, the next step is to build a yoga practice that suits your unique needs and lifestyle. A personalized approach allows you to choose poses, routines, and breathing techniques that resonate most with your body and mind. In this chapter, we'll discuss how to adapt yoga routines to fit individual needs, modify poses as necessary, and create a balanced practice that nurtures flexibility, strength, and mindfulness.

The Benefits of a Personalized Practice

Designing a practice tailored to your body and goals has multiple advantages:

- **Suits Your Body's Needs**: Each body is unique, with different flexibility levels, areas of tension, and preferences. Personalizing your practice ensures it supports your physical well-being.
- **Enhances Motivation and Enjoyment**: A routine built around your preferences can feel more enjoyable and sustainable over the long term.
- **Promotes Self-Discovery**: Adapting poses and routines encourages deeper self-

awareness and connection, as you tune in to what works best for you.

Adapting Routines to Personal Needs

Creating a routine that matches your current abilities and goals involves asking yourself the following:

1. **What are my primary goals?**: Determine if your focus is stress relief, increased flexibility, core strength, or another goal.
2. **What is my body's baseline?**: Take note of any areas of tightness, pain, or imbalance that need particular attention.
3. **What do I enjoy most about yoga?**: Identifying the poses, styles, or routines you find most rewarding can make it easier to create a practice that feels like "yours."

Modifying Poses for a Custom Fit

Adapting poses to your body's unique needs is key to a personalized practice. Here are some tips for modifying common poses:

- **Use Props**: Incorporate props like blocks, straps, and bolsters to enhance alignment and make poses more accessible.

- **Adjust for Flexibility**: If a pose is challenging due to flexibility, use a more supportive version, such as bending the knees in forward folds or using a block in standing poses.
- **Prioritize Alignment Over Depth**: For each pose, focus on correct alignment rather than trying to reach the "deepest" version of the pose. This approach prevents strain and supports long-term improvement.

Balancing Flexibility, Strength, and Mindfulness

A balanced practice incorporates these three pillars:

1. **Flexibility**: Stretching and gentle, mindful movement help increase flexibility over time. Including poses like Forward Fold and Low Lunge provides flexibility while releasing tension.
2. **Strength**: Build strength by including poses such as Plank, Warrior, and Chair Pose, which engage core and leg muscles.
3. **Mindfulness**: Keep your practice mindful by focusing on breath awareness and taking moments of stillness in poses like Child's Pose and Savasana.

Sample Personalized Practice Template

Here is a sample structure for creating a balanced practice:

1. **Warm-up**: Start with gentle stretches like Cat-Cow and Downward Dog.
2. **Flexibility Focus**: Include poses that target areas you want to make more flexible, such as Forward Fold or Reclined Butterfly.
3. **Strength Focus**: Add strength-building poses, choosing ones that align with your goals.
4. **Mindful Cooldown**: End with gentle restorative poses and a few minutes of deep breathing or meditation.

Summary of Chapter 14 Practices

This chapter emphasizes creating a practice that reflects your goals and preferences. By adjusting routines, modifying poses, and balancing flexibility, strength, and mindfulness, you can build a practice that feels personally meaningful and supports your well-being. The freedom to adapt your practice encourages continuous growth and a lasting connection with yoga.

Chapter 15: Maintaining Long-Term Health and Balance

Overview

As you complete this 30-day journey, sustaining your yoga practice can further enrich your life and deepen your connection to physical and mental well-being. This chapter provides strategies for maintaining a long-term yoga practice, tips for continuing to learn, and suggestions on how to expand your practice through community, resources, and advanced techniques.

Strategies for Continuing Your Practice

Consistency and enjoyment are key to keeping yoga a valuable part of your life. Here are some approaches to make yoga a lasting habit:

1. **Set Realistic Goals**: Identify what you want to achieve through ongoing practice, whether it's stress relief, flexibility, strength, or spiritual growth. Keep goals flexible to allow for your evolving interests.
2. **Build a Routine**: Choose a practice time that fits naturally into your day. For some, morning yoga sets a positive tone, while others may find evening practice relaxing.
3. **Practice Mindfulness**: Emphasize the quality of your practice over its length. A

mindful 10-minute practice can be as beneficial as a longer session.
4. **Mix it Up**: Incorporate new poses, routines, and themes into your practice to keep it engaging and adaptable to your current needs and interests.

Deepening Your Knowledge and Practice

Once you're comfortable with foundational poses and routines, continuing to learn can add depth to your practice:

- **Learn About Yoga Philosophy**: Exploring the philosophy behind yoga, such as the yamas (ethical principles) and niyamas (personal observances), can add a new dimension to your understanding.
- **Explore Advanced Breathing and Meditation Techniques**: Techniques like kapalabhati (breath of fire) or mindfulness meditation can complement and deepen your physical practice.
- **Focus on Alignment and Technique**: Advanced instruction can help refine poses, improve alignment, and prevent injury, adding both safety and depth to your practice.

Expanding Through Community and Resources

Connecting with others and utilizing resources can enrich your yoga experience:

1. **Group Classes**: Practicing in a class environment can provide valuable guidance, help correct alignment, and create a sense of community. Many find the shared energy in group settings inspiring.
2. **Online Resources**: Online classes and tutorials allow flexibility, letting you explore new styles, instructors, and themes at your own pace.
3. **Workshops and Retreats**: These immersive experiences offer intensive learning in areas like alignment, advanced poses, or yoga philosophy, ideal for those wanting a deeper commitment.

Exploring Advanced Poses (for Interested Practitioners)

For those who feel ready, advanced poses can challenge strength, flexibility, and mental focus. Examples include:

- **Arm Balances**: Poses like Crow Pose or Handstand build upper body strength and concentration.

- **Deep Backbends**: Advanced backbends such as Wheel or King Pigeon require both flexibility and strength, offering a rewarding challenge.
- **Inversions**: Inversions like Headstand or Shoulder Stand encourage confidence and provide new perspectives on movement and balance.

If you're interested in trying these poses, working with a qualified instructor for guidance is recommended to ensure proper technique.

This chapter guides you in creating a sustainable, enriching yoga practice that fits your unique lifestyle. By setting goals, expanding your learning, connecting with community, and incorporating advanced poses if desired, you can maintain balance and health through yoga for years to come. The journey of yoga continues, offering new insights and growth along the way.

Conclusion

Overview

Congratulations on completing this 30-day journey toward a more balanced, healthy, and resilient self through yoga! This conclusion will recap key takeaways, suggest resources for further study, and offer final encouragement to continue nurturing your practice.

Recap of Key Takeaways

Throughout this guide, you've explored the transformative benefits of yoga for managing stress, reducing pain, and overcoming fatigue. Here are some essential insights from each phase of your journey:

- **Stress Relief**: Through breathwork, mindfulness, and restorative poses, you learned how to calm the nervous system, ease mental strain, and release tension.
- **Pain Management**: Targeted yoga poses for areas prone to pain—such as the back, neck, shoulders, and hips—demonstrated how mindful movement can relieve discomfort and improve flexibility.
- **Fatigue Reduction**: By balancing energy-boosting morning routines with restful evening practices, you discovered how yoga can help regulate energy levels, allowing for

increased vitality during the day and deeper rest at night.

- **Personal Empowerment**: Through reflection, personalized routines, and goal-setting, you connected with yourself in a meaningful way, building awareness of your unique needs and fostering a deeper sense of self-care.

Resources for Further Study

Continuing your yoga journey is enriched by ongoing learning. Below are some recommended resources:

1. **Books**:
   - Light on Yoga by B.K.S. Iyengar – A classic guide on yoga postures and philosophy.
   - The Heart of Yoga by T.K.V. Desikachar – An accessible introduction to the principles and practice of yoga.
   - The Yamas & Niyamas by Deborah Adele – A study on yoga's ethical principles and personal observances.
2. **Apps**:
   - **YogaGlo** – Offers classes for all levels, including meditation and advanced techniques.

- o **Insight Timer** – A meditation app with guided sessions that complements your yoga practice.
  - o **Down Dog** – An adaptable yoga app with customizability for length, difficulty, and style.
3. **Online Yoga Communities**:
  - o **Yoga Alliance** – Connects you with certified teachers and classes and provides valuable resources.
  - o **Reddit (r/yoga)** – A supportive online forum where users discuss their yoga journeys, share tips, and offer guidance.

Encouragement to Continue the Journey

The path you've begun doesn't end here. Yoga is a lifelong practice of growth and self-discovery. As you move forward, remember:

- **Consistency is Key**: Practicing even a few minutes daily can maintain the physical, mental, and emotional benefits you've cultivated.
- **Listen to Your Body**: Allow your practice to evolve with your changing needs, and respect what your body needs in each moment.
- **Celebrate Small Wins**: Every session, no matter how brief, is a victory toward health and well-being.

Let this 30-day journey serve as the foundation for a lifetime of balance, resilience, and inner peace. The dedication you've shown to your practice is a gift to yourself that will keep giving, empowering you to face life's challenges with strength, calm, and joy. Thank you for embarking on this journey—here's to the next steps in your yoga path!

www.ingramcontent.com/pod-product-compliance
Lightning Source LLC
Chambersburg PA
CBHW051819250726
48659CB00005B/1578